**Teamwork in Pal**

# Teamwork in Palliative Care

## Fulfilling or Frustrating?

Edited by
Peter Speck

Former Health Care Chaplain

Honorary Senior Research Fellow
King's College London
Department of Palliative Care and Policy
Guy's King's and St Thomas' Medical School

Visiting Fellow
School of Psychology
Southampton University
UK

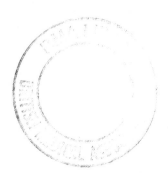

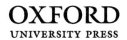

OXFORD
UNIVERSITY PRESS

# OXFORD
#### UNIVERSITY PRESS

Great Clarendon Street, Oxford OX2 6DP

Oxford University Press is a department of the University of Oxford.
It furthers the University's objective of excellence in research, scholarship,
and education by publishing worldwide in

Oxford New York

Auckland Cape Town Dar es Salaam Hong Kong Karachi
Kuala Lumpur Madrid Melbourne Mexico City Nairobi
New Delhi Shanghai Taipei Toronto

With offices in

Argentina Austria Brazil Chile Czech Republic France Greece
Guatemala Hungary Italy Japan South Korea Poland Portugal
Singapore Switzerland Thailand Turkey Ukraine Vietnam

Oxford is a registered trade mark of Oxford University Press
in the UK and in certain other countries

Published in the United States
by Oxford University Press Inc., New York

© Oxford University Press 2006
© Chapter 6/Noreen Ramsay

The moral rights of the author have been asserted
Database right Oxford University Press (maker)

First published 2006
Reprinted 2007 (with corrections)

A catalogue record for this title is available from the British Library

Library of Congress Cataloging in Publication Data
Teamwork in palliative care : fulfilling or frustrating? / edited by Peter Speck.
Includes bibliographical references and index.
ISBN-13: 978-0-19-856774-5 (alk. paper)
1. Palliative treatment. 2. Hospice care. I. Speck, Peter W.
[DNLM: 1. Palliative Care–methods. 2. Palliative Care–organization & administration.
3. Patient Care Team–organization & administration. WB 310 T2535 2006]
R726.8.T43 2006 616'.029—dc22 2006017844

Typeset by SPI Publisher Services, Pondicherry, India
Printed in Great Britain
on acid-free paper by
Biddles Ltd., King's Lynn, Norfolk

ISBN 978-0-19-856774-5

10 9 8 7 6 5 4 3 2

# Dedication

In memory of Frances Sheldon who modelled and taught the importance of multidisciplinary teamwork to so many.

# Acknowledgements

Acknowledgements are due to various people. First a warm and sincere acknowledgement to those teams that I have worked in, or led, who enabled me to learn so much about the ways we interact with each other and the skills needed to develop and maintain a healthy functioning team. Secondly to the other authors within this book who generously agreed to contribute to this work and to debate with me some of the issues we have explored here. Thirdly to my wife and family who have always offered support, encouragement and necessary distractions, and various individuals who have probably not realized how much they have contributed over the years to shaping my own development and understanding of organizational and team dynamics—including Anton Obholtzer and Vega Roberts of the Tavistock Clinic London, The Royal Free Hospital Palliative Care Team and the many students and staff groups I have taught, supervised or consulted over the years. I am also appreciative of the team at Oxford University Press who have helped bring the vision of such a text into reality—especially Georgia Pinteau and Catherine Barnes; and to Noreen Ramsay and Routledge publishers for permission to reproduce the chapter 'Sitting close to death—a palliative care unit' within Chapter 6 of this volume.

I am also honoured that Professor Mary Vachon has been willing to write the Foreword to this book.

Peter Speck

# Contents

# Contents

# List of contributors

**Abraham Adunsky MD**
Director of Geriatric Department
Sheba Medical Center
Senior Lecturer
Tel Aviv University
Tel HaShomer 52621
Israel

**Michaela Bercovitch MD**
Research and Information Coordinator
Tel Ha Shomer Oncological Hospice
Sheba Medical Center
Lecturer in Palliative Care
Tel Aviv University
Tel HaShomer 52621
Israel

**Professor Ian Maddocks**
Emeritus Professor
Flinders University
Adelaide
South Australia

**David Oliviere**
Director of Education and Training
St Christopher's Hospice
51–59 Lawrie Park Road
London SE26 6DZ
UK

**Dr Noreen Ramsay**
Psychiatrist and Ceramic Artist
c/o Taylor & Francis (Routledge)
27 Church Road
Hove, Sussex BN3 2FA
UK

**Professor Malcolm Payne**
Director of Psycho-social and
Spiritual Care
St Christopher's Hospice
51–59 Lawrie Park Road
London SE26 6DZ
UK

**Dr Iain Lawrie**
Specialist Registrar in Palliative
Medicine
The Leeds Teaching Hospitals NHS
Trust
Great George Street
Leeds LS1 3EX
UK

**Professor Mari Lloyd-Williams MD,
FRCP, MRCGP, MMedSci, ILTM**
Professor/Honorary Consultant in
Palliative Medicine
Academic Palliative and Supportive
Care Studies Group (APSCSG)
Division of Primary Care
School of Population, Community
and Behavioural Sciences
University of Liverpool
2nd Floor Whelan Building
Brownlow Hill
Liverpool L69 3GB
UK

**Dr Bobbie Farsides**
Professor of Clinical and Biomedical Ethics
Brighton and Sussex Medical School
University of Sussex
Brighton, Sussex BN1 9PX
UK

**Professor Jonathan Montgomery**
Professor of Health Care Law
School of Law
Southampton University, Highfield,
Southampton SO17 1BJ
UK

**Barbara Monroe**
Chief Executive
St Christopher's Hospice
51–59 Lawrie Park Road
London SE26 6DZ
UK

**Peter Speck**
(Former Health Care Chaplain)
Honorary Senior Research Fellow
King's College London
Department of Palliative Care,
Policy and Rehabilitation
Guy's, King's and St Thomas' Medical School
Western Education Centre
Cutcombe Road, Denmark Hill
London SE5 9RJ

and

Visiting Fellow, School of Psychology
Southampton University
Highfield
Southampton SO17 1BJ
UK

# Foreword

Having been researching, writing and lecturing in the field of occupational stress in health care professionals for more than thirty years and having done one of the first studies of stress in palliative care staff, it was with a great deal of enthusiasm that I accepted Peter Speck's offer to write the Foreword for this important book on *Teamwork in Palliative Care*.

In the early days of hospice, Dr. Balfour Mount quoted Dame Cicely Saunders as saying "if you say that you work on a team, then you have to be prepared to show your battle scars." My own early work in the field with my colleagues, the study I did exploring the stress of almost 600 caregivers from around the world (1), and more recent review chapters continue to find that teams are a major source of our stress, the place where our stress is often manifest and the place we turn to for help in coping with the stress of our daily work. This book sheds light on these and other topics and raises new questions. It has been said that when the light is shed it illuminates some of the shadows and dark corners that are often left unexplored. This book serves to offer such illumination.

Peter Speck raises the question of whether teams are the best way in which to carry out palliative care. Despite everyone "knowing" that it is the only approach to take, he and Barbara Monroe show that the evidence is not there. Good palliative care makes a difference, but is this difference primarily because of well-functioning teams or could it be equally well delivered by sufficiently resourced individuals? – a fascinating question and one which will no doubt cause consternation to some readers.

The authors draw on current literature, with reference to earlier works as appropriate, and use clinical examples to get the reader thinking about a number of deceptively basic questions such as what is a group and what is a team? How do they differ? How does leadership evolve and devolve in a variety of situations? How does the setting effect the team? What about leadership and followers-issues of power and authority? What is it really like to be with dying people?

Oliviere makes specific suggestions for really involving the patient and family as equal partners in the decision-making process and in planning for care, pointing out that care is often designed for the care providers rather than primarily for the needs of the patient and family. A palliative care nurse came to visit a client with whom I was working. The nurse had a list of questions for the patient to complete for the team's use. The patient's response was "even my oncologist, whom I have known for years, has never asked me such questions; I am not sure why you need this information". For what purpose is the team gathering information and what are the ethical issues involved in obtaining such information? The question is raised about who users would choose as their "team of choice" at various points in the cancer trajectory. Specific suggestions are given regarding involving users in collaborative roles, moving beyond simply giving lip service to the "patient and family as the unit of care".

Issues of team roles, with flexible boundaries, maintaining a healthy team, and team building, communication and training are dealt with well. So too are the ethical and legal issues involved in areas such as differences of opinion within the team about specific treatments and issues such as euthanasia and physician assisted suicide. The authors suggest that in a healthy team there will be room for disagreement and give specific suggestions for handling conflicts. They also strongly suggest that, rather than team members leaving the team if they do not agree with the ethical decision making of other team members, they should stay and hold the contrary view giving space for differing views within the team context. Interesting to see how this could hold up in practice.

The issue of the values of team members is addressed, "whether the experience we have at work is fulfilling or frustrating will depend to a large extent on how these values blend to form a team culture and match, or clash with our own personal values." This discussion is particularly important in view of the fact that Maslach and colleagues (2) have found that congruence with one's value system is one of the most important factors in protecting individuals from burnout, along with a sense of community. Teams may or may not give this sense of community.

Peter Speck notes that central to the meeting of the total pain needs of those whom we serve is the importance of "the nature of the relationships that exist and the trust and respect engendered between those involved in providing consultation or hands on care to, and with, the person who is ill." This requires trust within the team. This may not be easy as the shadow sides of each of us as individuals comes with us as we come into our team roles. Chapter 6 provides valuable insight into the dynamics of a team, as both individuals and team members, surfacing issues, such as conscious and unconscious process, defences against emotion, and "chronic niceness" as a way of dealing with primitive and powerful feelings which are "not nice". These are issues which have interested me for the decades I have worked in the field, and they seldom find their way into discussion in the literature.

*Teamwork in Palliative Care* comes at an important point of transition in the palliative care movement. Both Derek Doyle (3) and Michael Kearney (4) warned about the move from palliative care to palliative medicine many years ago. This book helps to keep the care within the palliative care team, while recognizing that we are moving into the future.

Mary L.S. Vachon , RN, PhD
Psychotherapist and Consultant in Private Practice,
Professor,
Departments of Psychiatry and Public Health Science
University of Toronto

## References

1. Vachon MLS. (1987) Occupational stress in the care of the critically ill, dying and bereaved. Washington, DC: Hemisphere.
2. Maslach C, Schaufeli WB, Leiter MP. (2001) Job burnout. *Annual Reviews Psychology.* 52: 397–422.
3. Doyle D. (1992) Have we looked beyond the physical and psychosocial? Journal of Pain and Symptom Management. 7: 302–311
4. Kearney M. (1992) Palliative medicine-just another specialty? Palliative Medicine. 6: 41.

# 1

# Introduction

*Peter Speck*

It has been acknowledged from the early days of palliative care that teamwork is an essential component. The needs of people diagnosed with life-threatening disease will vary greatly over time and make a variety of demands on the skills of the caregivers who are involved with the patient's journey. It is rarely possible for any one professional to provide for all these needs. Therefore, the skills of others are needed if a holistic approach is to be maintained. This has been clear since the beginning of the modern hospice movement as reflected in David Clark's selection from the letters of the late Cicely Saunders.

When a patient told Cicely Saunders 'all of me is wrong' or another said 'it was *all* pain' it became increasingly apparent that the required response included a breadth of vision for its understanding and huge versatility in its alleviation. As early as 1964 the concept of 'total pain' had been described in its full form and was taken to include physical symptoms, mental distress, social problems, and emotional difficulties. The emerging field of terminal care had now been furnished with one of its most important and enduring concepts.... (Clark 2002, p. 9).

To deliver care across such a wide range of need, including the spiritual, would require more skill than one individual alone could deliver, in spite of Dame Cicely herself spanning three professions and having a devout spiritual life. The need for people with a variety of skills to work together was also being recognized and, with the help of the 'total pain' model, a more integrated approach was adopted. Forty years later, how these additional skills, knowledge and insights are brought into play depends on many factors, but central is the nature of the relationships that exist, and the trust and respect engendered between those involved in providing consultation or hands-on care to, and with, the person who is ill. If the patient is not to be confused by conflicting advice, or their care compromised by the range of different people they meet in the course of their illness journey, there needs to be coordination and collaboration. Teams offer a way of achieving this, but they exist in a variety of forms. While this book focuses on the importance of teams within palliative care, we believe the thoughts and reflections are also applicable to a variety of care settings. The authors represent palliative care work in a variety of countries, and we are now aware of how many parts of the world are seeking to acquire palliative care skills and develop services. It is envisaged that, just as palliative care is a global issue, this book will also have a global appeal to newly forming as well as long-established palliative care teams.

As palliative care has developed, so have different styles of working. There has been an evolutionary process dictated by several factors including vision, funding, availability of skilled people and an increased recognition of the need for such a service—not least for those with non-cancerous conditions. In some cases, palliative care has been provided by a lone worker supported, one hopes, by a 'back home' team of colleagues who may not necessarily be experienced in palliative care. This person may work out in the community or within a large general acute hospital and can find it quite difficult to establish their role, demonstrate their expertise or meet the expectations of those making referrals if they have to cover a large geographical area.

In other settings, there may be a collection of professionals who agree to work together and share their skills in the best interests of the patient and family. The composition of this group will depend very much on the resources available to those responsible for the provision of care—in terms of both finance and personal skill. It may not be feasible for that group to form itself into a clearly designated team immediately, and so a loose 'confederation' may be formed of like-minded individuals, as a transitional stage of development. Whether or not this collection of people will later constitute an effective team will be determined, to a large extent, by the clarity of their understanding of the task, and the degree to which they can each own it and collaborate with an agreed form of leadership. The style and quality of the leadership will affect many aspects of their working life and the extent to which the sum total of their combined work is greater than their individual contributions. Individual personalities, and the interactions which occur within the organization in which they work, will determine both the effectiveness with which they provide care *and* the amount of personal and professional satisfaction they receive. This book will examine the process of forming and sustaining a healthy and effective team.

The nature of palliative care is such that the work itself can affect the caregiver as well as the patient and family. This may be a side effect of the relationship that develops between the patient and the professional caregiver. It might also be because the caregiver is affected by the re-awakening of some unresolved conflict in their own life which has been triggered by the interaction with the patient or family. Appropriate support is therefore vital on both an individual and a team basis. Equally the caregiver may be affected by the interpersonal and interteam dynamic created within the organization within which their team is located. The element of uncertainty that seems to arise regularly within both the National Health Service (NHS) and the charity sector, because of financial pressures and organizational change, also contributes to stress and anxiety for staff at all levels. We cannot assume that all teams will continue to work within in-patient units since structural changes may dictate new patterns of palliative care provision and therefore new forms of team working (see Chapter 13 of this volume). Because of this uncertainty, and the complexity of the endeavour, teamwork in palliative care can oscillate between fulfilment and frustration on both a personal and a professional level.

Palliative care is concerned with the provision of high quality care to vulnerable people, many of whom may be approaching the end of their life. Those providing that care are involved in a process which includes diagnosis, assessment, treatment and care options, choices, responding to crises, etc. which occur along a time scale from diagnosis to death—and, for the family, into bereavement. This is often described as a 'care pathway' along which interventions take place in an integrated way (Ellershaw and Wilkinson 2003). Along this time line, many people will become involved, each with a particular contribution to the process of care. Some will be invited to advise on a particular problem or aspect of care, or to make a specific intervention in that care, and afterwards will go away. Others will already be part of the palliative care team but with a specific contribution to make from the insights and expertise of their own discipline. These latter will be more integrated into the ongoing life of the team and have a more direct accountability for their contributions.

Some of the steps in the care process (interventions) will happen in isolation from others and will always carry the possibility of breakdown in the process, especially because of failures in communication often in terms of expectations of each other. Each person or group making a contribution to care will be involved in the processes relevant to their own specialty, and together these will contribute to the wider system or organization in which they work. For the system to work well, and seamless care to be experienced by the patient and family, there needs to be a strong sense of working together in order to achieve individual, group and organizational objectives. We shall discuss the key role held by leaders in creating a teamwork attitude which reminds people that everyone is interdependent and successful care requires people to cooperate with each other. One factor that helps people to cooperate is a shared set of values.

## The importance of values

When people come to work, they wish to engage with activities that are consistent with the values they hold. Values are what people believe to be

3

right, wrong, good, desirable, moral, etc. These values have developed in a variety of ways including: family life, education, belief system (religious and otherwise), peer group relationships and professional identity, and can affect how we function at work. Thus if someone holds beliefs that ending the life of another is always morally wrong then, as a health care worker, they would not usually want to be involved in terminating a pregnancy or aiding someone's suicide, because it conflicted with their values. The various professions will also, in their codes of practice, enshrine some core values that the profession would wish members to uphold. Teamwork depends to a certain extent on people being able to subscribe to a *shared* set of values which reinforce the team way of working and reduce the likelihood of clashes with personal values. These values might include the following.

- *The importance of working together to achieve the aim.* This means that if something goes wrong, you look at the 'whole team' process and not just an individual. Focusing on the individual implies that it is the individual's not the team's performance that is important.
- As with the patient, so also *each team member deserves respect.* There may be different levels of responsibility and accountability within a team, but this should not imply that some people are worth more than others.
- Valuing of *open and honest communication* arises out of respect and implies an attitude of listening to each other and developing an understanding of the other person's point of view.
- Information can be power, and in true teamwork there needs to be *open access to information* so that some team members are not disempowered. It is hard to cooperate if information you need is being withheld, but there are issues about what people 'need to know' to do their job and people do not necessarily need to know everything.
- To *value the people you work with and attend to the dynamic processes* which develop as a way of fostering mutual respect and achieving the desired outcome for the work of the team.

Whether the experience we have at work is fulfilling or frustrating will depend to a large extent on how these values blend to form a team culture and match, or clash, with our own personal values (see Chapter 11 of this volume). If they match, we are more likely to engage with others in achieving common goals. If they do not match, we may engage in activities designed more to fulfil our own goals, often described as 'off-task' activity.

## Varieties of team

Teamwork can enable people to work toward common goals, pool their expertise in the best interests of the patient and the service, and provide a forum for problem solving—ethical and otherwise. They can also be of benefit by sharing the burden of the work and providing space within which people can grow and develop. There are many adjectives found preceding the word team—multi-professional, multidisciplinary, interdisciplinary, project, senior management, etc.—all attracting differing opinions as to their benefits and burdens. Because of the centrality of team working in palliative care, we must enhance awareness and understanding of the things that happen within teams in order that they develop in healthy and creative ways, and be able to recognize when there are difficulties and have strategies to deal with them. This book seeks to address these important issues because effective team working can enhance the quality of care received by patient and family, and support the caregiver in fulfilling that aim.

The key benefit of team working is perhaps best seen when patients and families are able to share a wide range of needs and vulnerabilities as they reveal different things to different team members. Trust and confidence grow as the patient sees that the team can contain distress and bring the fragmented aspects of care together, respond to them in a holistic way and enable the patient to access the wide range of skills which are held within the team.

At present there is little written about this crucial and central aspect of specialist palliative care, apart from journal articles and chapters in more generic textbooks. We hope that this text will further develop the integrated approach envisaged in the NICE guidance *Improving Supportive and Palliative Care for Adults with Cancer*, and be of benefit to those who offer palliative care in a variety of settings and understandings of the word 'team'.

This book explores the different aspects of team working as they apply to palliative care. How does a team come into being and what different formats are there? How might the users of the service contribute to the life of the team and the service offered? What are the difficulties and frustrations encountered in developing and maintaining such teams? Because palliative care is provided by a variety of different disciplines, what models of working and styles of leadership have developed? How are power and authority handled within the team setting? Teams do not just happen and so the importance of team building, training, support, attention to group process and stress management to protect the mental health of the team will be explored. By its very nature, end-of-life care and palliative care engage with many of the thorny ethical issues in care. It is important, therefore, to address the effect of working across professional boundaries, and with people outside of a professional role, in relation to consent, autonomy, confidentiality, decision making within teams and the legal implications of such team working. The book concludes with the important question—do we know if teams *are* the most effective way of providing care?

These different questions are addressed by a variety of authors, all of whom are experts in the field with many years experience of palliative care. We hope that readers will find this a useful and helpful guide to reappraising the importance of collaborative teamwork and enhance their understanding of the teams within which they currently work.

## References

Ellershaw J and Wilkinson S (2003). *Care of the Dying: A Pathway to Excellence*. Oxford University Press, Oxford.

Clark D (2002). *Cicely Saunders—Founder of the Hospice Movement. Selected Letters 1959–1999*. Oxford University Press, Oxford.

# 2

# Team or group—spot the difference

*Peter Speck*

The ability to work well within a team is frequently seen as an essential personal attribute in recruitment advertisements. Within the health care setting, team working is frequently advocated as the preferred style because it is assumed that teams deliver more than individuals and provides a panacea for performance and motivational difficulties. It is questionable if this is the case. There can often be a gap between the expected outcome and reality, as evidenced in the 1890s when Max Ringelmann, a French agricultural engineer, showed that a group pulling on a rope exerted approximately 75 per cent of the force that these individuals could produce when working separately. In other words, there can be a tendency for individuals to expend less effort when working as a member of a group than as an individual (Kravitz and Martin 1986). Teamwork, however, is a fashionable term and, as Belbin (2000) points out, has begun to replace the former term group work, and begs the question: is there really any difference?

## Groups

Our personal identity is formed and shaped as a result of our interaction with other people as well as the expression of our basic genetic makeup. We, therefore, seek out and develop formal and informal social groups and networks in both our private and our working life which supplement the relationship we already have within our family unit. We may therefore belong to a variety of groups which meet for a range of activities.

The social psychologists Sherif and Sherif (1969) believed that the key component for a group was the *presence of a social structure*, generally in the form of status and role relationships. For example, within a family, the group has an implicit social structure since each family member has well-defined relationships with each other and normally there are clear roles and differences of status. Harré and Lamb (1986) offer a definition of a group as being 'two or more people who are interacting with one another, who share a set of common goals and norms which direct their activities, and who develop a set of roles and a network of affective relationships'.

Groups tend to be classified in a variety of ways usually related to their purpose:

- *Informal or social*: where the purpose is less precise but understood and accepted by all involved, e.g. the darts group who meet at the public house, holiday groups, social groups in the coffee lounge or supporters at a sporting event.

- *Formal*: formed for a precise purpose, usually with rules and regulations which may prescribe behaviour expected of members as well as how people move into or out of the group, e.g. golf club, committee meetings, conferences, annual general meetings or project groups.

- *Psychological*: groups which are dependent upon people interacting with each other, being aware of each other and perceiving that they belong, e.g. a therapeutic group or self-help group.

- Groups may also be formed on the basis of
  the beliefs and values of the members—as with religious or political groups the expertise of members—professional bodies, mutual interest—as with hobbies and interests.

Groups may have a short life, as in the case of a party gathering or waiting to board a delayed aircraft at the airport, or be long lasting such as with a school community, a religious community or patients sharing the life of a long-stay hospital ward. A group can cross cultural and national boundaries in a way that brings into focus the importance of communication if the group is to retain any cohesiveness.

From this recognition of the variety of groups that we may enter and leave during our personal and professional life, we may abstract some general characteristics, as outlined in Table 2.1.

**Table 2.1** Some common group characteristics

- The development of a collective identity which is based on the circumstances and environment in which people find themselves. For example, as a spinal injury patient in a long-stay unit.
- The ability of members to communicate with each other.
- Some shared aims and objectives. In the airport example, this might be eventually to board their plane and arrive safely at their destination.
- Developing structures and roles. Leadership may begin to emerge in that some people may assert themselves to try and influence the outcome and other people.
- Norms and rules may be formed, adhered to or flouted. Behaviour may be modified by individual members in the presence of the wider group, or variations of behaviour may be sanctioned by the group, or emerging leadership, because of the circumstances. In the event of a fire in a public place, for example, the norm of not opening emergency exits will be ignored to enable escape from the building, and the norm of riding in the lift would be resisted because of the increased risk.

The size of a group can vary enormously, from four or five people, to several hundred, or until its size reaches that of a crowd, or even a unruly mob. Once the group size reaches crowd proportions, it is difficult to identify any real interaction between all of the individuals who often see themselves as individuals *within* a group rather than members *of* a group. This echoes the description of a group offered by Schein (1988) as:

.... Any number of people who (1) interact with one another, (2) are psychologically aware of one another, and (3) perceive themselves to be a group.

In the process of our life, we will move in and out of many groups because of geographical moves, changes of allegiance, change of job and changes of group because of interest or age. As a result, we will acquire skills and experience to help us engage with the process of joining, belonging and leaving. We will also acquire positive and negative memories as we experience the pleasures and the pains of sharing, communicating, and the inclusive/exclusive nature of some group activities. When we enter work for the first time, or a new work group, we will draw on a range of experiences to encourage or discourage us as we seek to engage with the new people. The same mixture of feelings can be aroused if we are invited, or recruited, to join a small group in order to participate in addressing a particular task or developing a service through the formation of a team. The influence of early experiences of groups and teams is a theme we shall return to later when we review some of the effects of team dynamics on team members.

## Teams

In many ways, a team is a group of people brought together, from within or outside of the organization, for a specific purpose or task. In working to achieve the task, it is expected that members will work interdependently and take some ownership for the outcome.

There is tendency to use the terms *groups* and *teams* interchangeably. However, Belbin (2000) questions this interchangeability and believes it important to clarify their use in order to protect the special characteristics of teams. He believes there are several factors which distinguish between teams and groups. These include size, selection of membership, leadership, style and spirit or ethos.

In particular, issues of leadership and style are at the fore and show themselves as pulling in opposite directions. The quintessential feature of a small well-balanced team is that leadership is shared or rotates. As critical issues arise, different individuals come to the fore and make their special contribution. In the typical group, a very different situation prevails. The leadership stays unchanged in spite of the changing focus of the work, for solo leaders are not easily challenged or displaced. When solo leaders gain their ascendancy in a group, they nearly always set out to standardize policies. They impose their own particular style and preferences on others. Dissenters are unwelcome. Inner tensions are released through external expression, while any lingering hostility is now deflected towards outsiders. The sequence of events then is that large groups typically throw up solo leaders. (Belbin 2000, p.15)

The popularity of teams is seen in part as a side effect of the increasing preoccupation with empowerment and self-management and leads some authors to ask 'why do we want teams?' If teams are simply a convenient way to group a lot of people, who used to work under several supervisors, under one manager then do not bother, says Holpp (1997). However, Holpp also states that if teams can truly take ownership of the work and provide the kind of close-up knowledge that is not available elsewhere, then full speed ahead. Sometimes organizations are not always sure whether they have teams or groups of people working together. It is certainly true to say that any group of people who do not know they are a team cannot be one. To become a team, a group of individuals needs to have a strong common purpose (primary task) and to work towards that purpose rather than individually. They also need to believe that they will achieve more by cooperation by than working individually (Cane 1996).

Having a clear primary task which is 'owned' by each member of the team is central to the transition of group to team. How you define the task will have great significance in how the team works and is an important factor contributing to team effectiveness and member satisfaction, as illustrated in Box 2.1.

The best way of differentiating between groups and teams is in terms of size, leadership and task. Groups can comprise any number of people, whereas teams will usually contain not more than 12 people, and frequently less. The style of leadership can also be a key differentiator, with a small well-balanced team having a leadership that is shared and may rotate according to the activity focused on at any particular time in order to best achieve the team's task or aim. Within larger groups, the leadership tends to emerge out of the group as solo leadership, which sometimes may be contested by other group members.

## Varieties of team

Some teams are *permanent* groupings of people who have a responsibility for a particular ongoing set of operations or processes. Their membership is usually made up of people within the same department such as the hospital post room or the radiotherapy department. In addition to their day to day work, the team may carry responsibility for monitoring their effectiveness and ways of working to ensure the smooth running of their department. They will also be expected to be accountable for improving their work processes and meeting targets.

## Box 2.1 THE EFFECT OF HOW WE UNDERSTAND THE TASK

It is possible to think of an organization in terms of a set of interdependent systems which interact with each other to provide the product or aim of the organization. This is termed an 'open system' which is one which absorbs 'inputs' in the form of raw material, finance, people or information. These are then 'processed' to provide a variety of 'outputs' in terms of goods or services. The system will usually have subsystems which all need to collaborate if the desired outcome is to be achieved. Therefore, feedback is crucial to the open system model in order that resources and priorities can be properly allocated.

Figure 2.1 represents an 'open system'. Let us suppose it is a diagrammatic representation of a sausage factory. At point 1, we have the input of raw materials: the meat, bread, herbs, skins, etc. Within the organization we have subsystems which undertake the conversion of the raw materials into the end-product or output of tasty and succulent sausages. We also have systems which focus on marketing and packaging, as well as distribution. The various boundaries within the systems are managed so that raw meat does not turn up in the marketing department or labels turn up in the processing section. All work harmoniously together to produce the desired product.

If we transfer this model to palliative care, we *could* suggest that the input is the receipt of people who have life-threatening conditions. The output could be described as dead people. If this is accepted as true, then the primary aim of the organization (palliative care unit or team) is to convert dying live people into dead people, and to continue to do that every day of every year. Clearly this is a parody of what palliative care is concerned with, but it illustrates the way in which our understanding of the primary task will influence how we do the work and the effect that work will have upon us. In reality, the input is people with life-threatening conditions and the output will be that some of them will have died. However, a lot will have been discharged home having had their symptoms and condition alleviated, or received help with rehabilitation needs. All should be receiving care which will enhance their quality of life until such time as they die, whether that be in the short or long term. This understanding of the primary task means that the staff take up their role in a different way which will not render them immune from stress and emotional load, but will provide a degree of job satisfaction and reward arising from their ability to support patients in this last stage of their life, drawing upon the skills and abilities of other team members to achieve the 'best' outcome.

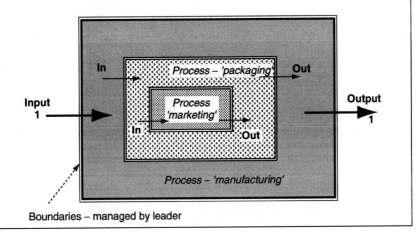

11

New developments or restructuring of work within the organization might be undertaken by a project team. This team may come from outside the organization, but if from within, it will usually have a *temporary* structure and comprise people from several departments who are brought together because of their particular skills to complete the project brief. During the time of the project, they will be responsible for its design, development and completion. At the end of the project, they will cease to be a team and will either leave the organization, if an external team, or return to their original departments if recruited from within the organization. In organizational terminology, they are often described as a cross-functional team because they consist of members from different functional areas of the organization who come together solely to work on the allocated task and to complete it in the allotted time span.

Teams may also be classified according to management type. Some teams will have a manager who is responsible for, and has authority over, the team's actions. Alternatively, a team may be self-managed, or self-directing. In this situation, all the members are jointly responsible for executing the process and completing the task. To succeed, such teams need to have a major commitment to the importance of teamwork. They also require sufficient experience and understanding to take responsibility for managing their own working practice. Often such teams will have acquired sufficient understanding and skill to be able to 'fill in' or help each other to assist the entire team to function effectively when individual colleagues are under pressure. For example, a degree of computer literacy may be acquired, or counselling skills training, to enable others to share a sudden increase in workload which might otherwise fall to one individual to cope with. This model or style is close to that seen in some specialist palliative care teams who have been together long enough to have acquired the necessary trust, skill and respect for each other's disciplines to be able to transcend boundaries when the immediate needs of the task or patient require them to do.

It is possible to identify other types of team within a health care setting, and staff at various levels within the organization may find themselves moving into and out of a variety of structures during their working life. These might include the Middle Management team, Change Management team, Service development team, Major Incident Response team, Executive Management team, and so on. Within palliative care in particular, we experience a variety of understandings and expressions of teamwork, with the most common being multidisciplinary and interdisciplinary.

### Multidisciplinary teams

Multidisciplinary teams are common within medical settings where individual members are primarily known by their professional identity. Their affiliation to the team is of secondary importance. Information within such a team is usually via the medical record, each professional adding to the record details of their interaction with the patient. The leadership of such a team is usually held by the highest ranking person which, in hospital life, is frequently a medical consultant. In many ways, the individuals act as a federation and the level in interaction is not necessarily expected to be very high. Thus a chaplain or a physiotherapist will be asked to see a patient with a view to making an assessment or an intervention. They will then report back to the multidisciplinary team at a team meeting or via the medical record, but there may not be any further integration into the ongoing life of that clinical team. In some ways, they are like the slightly exploded pieces of a pie-chart in that each person has a defined role in the assessment and provision of care for the patient, but will often make their contribution in seeming isolation from the others.

It is interesting to see that this is close to the model described in the NICE (UK) guidance for improving supportive and palliative care (NICE 2004) in which they define the multidisciplinary team as:

A group of health and social care professionals from a range of disciplines who meet regularly to discuss and agree plans of treatment and care for people with a particular type of cancer or problem, or in a particular location. Includes primary care teams, site-specific cancer teams and specialist palliative care teams (p. 200).

The Key Recommendation 3 of the NICE guidance manual advocates that:

Each multidisciplinary team or service should implement processes to ensure effective inter-professional communication within teams and between them and other service providers with whom the patient has contact. Mechanisms should be developed to promote continuity of care, which might include the nomination of a person to take on the role of 'key worker' for individual patients (p. 7).

This key recommendation is close to the understanding of interdisciplinary teamwork, described below. It seems to illustrate the way in which, within palliative care, one finds a spectrum of styles of team working which often relate to the place where care is delivered, the evolutionary stage of the specialist palliative care programme and the resources available. Within specialist palliative care, there is an emphasis on a holistic approach to the patient and the care offered, and a desire to provide a seamless pattern of care for the patient to maximize the quality of life for that patient.

The focus of palliative care is well described by the World Health Organization (2002) as:

... the active holistic care of patients with advanced, progressive illness. Management of pain and other symptoms and provision of psychological, social and spiritual support is paramount. The goal of palliative care is achievement of the best quality of life for patients and their families. Many aspects of palliative care are also applicable earlier in the course of the illness in conjunction with other treatments.

To achieve the best quality of life for patients and families, there needs to be good coordination in terms of care planning and delivery of that care over time. To increase the chances of this happening, many specialist palliative care teams move from a multidisciplinary model to an interdisciplinary one where there is a much higher degree of inter-relatedness between the various members of the team.

### Interdisciplinary teams

The hallmarks of an interdisciplinary team are described by Cummings (1998) where 'the identity of the team supersedes individual personal identities. Members share information and work interdependently together to develop goals. Leadership is shared among team members depending on the task at hand. Because the team is the vehicle of action, the interaction process is vital to success' (p. 19).

The interaction within the team is required to produce the final product, in this case high quality holistic care for patients and families, with the team achieving more than the sum total of the individuals involved. The interaction can have the effect of enabling individual practitioners to learn from each other and so extend and enhance their own skills, while acknowledging the limits of their ability. For example, a doctor or nurse who has developed a wider understanding of spiritual care may feel more able to discuss existential and spiritual issues with patients who want to explore these areas. There may come a point where the doctor or nurse recognizes that the conversation is moving to the edges of their own personal experience, or their ability to assist the patient, and would then involve another team member more skilled or specialized in providing spiritual/existential support.

In other words, there will be limits to the extent to which team members can 'cover' for each other, but there may also be great scope for team members to offer general patient support with a range of needs until it is clear another resource person is required. That resource person (e.g. spiritual care provider/ chaplain) may then work directly with the patient or may offer support to the team member who has the primary relationship with the patient and support them in continuing their exploration of issues with the patient. Within an interdisciplinary team, there is a high level of mutual accountability which will require good documentation, effective communication skills and trust, and clarity and commitment to the primary task, in order to ensure continuity of care. Failure to achieve this can result in confused, delayed or clumsy referrals to team colleagues and reduced quality of care for the patient.

Interdisciplinary working can be very creative for problem solving and is especially relevant to specialist palliative care where ethical concerns abound. However, it is important that the contributions of individual members of the team are respected and valued. When we examine some of the issues relating to team dynamics, we shall see that feeling respected and valued is a key component of effective team working (Chapter 7, this volume).

Whether the palliative care team operates in a multidisciplinary or interdisciplinary way, the composition of the team is very important. For both practical and philosophical reasons, opinions vary as to who should be a member of the team.

## Membership

Within palliative care, the development of a skilled resource may be an evolutionary process. In the early stages, there may be limited financial resources and the service may need to rely on a single individual working within an acute hospital setting, a primary care team, or as a charity-supported worker seeking to develop an understanding of palliative care within a given geographical area. Over time, it may be possible to recruit others and begin the formation of a team of people having the same or different professional identities. If the service continues to develop and to establish a variety of ways of providing the service (in-patient beds, out-patient clinic, home care, rehabilitation, education, the use of volunteers, etc.), there will come a point at which decisions need to be made regarding team membership: how will those members relate to each other and who will lead them?

If we consider the acute hospital setting, the patient may have his/her palliative care needs assessed and met by a palliative care specialist who enters the multidisciplinary ward-based team to offer advice to those with the primary responsibility for clinical care. The palliative care input may be provided by a specialist nurse or doctor who is a sole appointee to a hospital at the early stages of developing a service. The input may, however, be from a member of a well-established interdisciplinary palliative care team based within the hospital or within a local specialist palliative care unit. The membership, philosophy and style of leadership may be very different in each of these teams.

If membership of the interdisciplinary specialist palliative care team is related to the needs of the patient and family, then the team may comprise a range of people. Potential team members could be:

The patient and family
Nursing staff
Chaplain/spiritual care provider
Occupational therapist
Dietitian
Complementary therapists
Medical staff

Social worker
Physiotherapist
Pharmacist
Volunteers
Counsellor/psychologist

Cummings (1998) provides a description of many of these roles. However, it is important that team members do not rely on second-hand descriptions of other people's roles and functions as they can easily lead to stereotyping. Within any team that is forming, as well as during its ongoing life, members should explore each other's roles and develop an understanding of the role, and the person in the role, in order to begin to appreciate and value what they might bring to the life of the team and the service they offer. Much tension can be created within teams if people continue to operate at the level of assumptions, and possible prejudice, about each other and do not undertake this essential exploration. Difference can be a creative and vital ingredient in the formation of a team.

In writing about palliative care ethics, Randall and Downie (1996) acknowledge the importance of team work in palliative care, but suggest that we need to recognize the intrinsic and extrinsic membership of that team. They state that the concept of the multidisciplinary team has always been central to the philosophy of palliative care, and that the knowledge and skills of many health care professionals are essential if the intrinsic and extrinsic aims of palliative care are to be met. Specialist palliative care teams within in-patient units tend to consist of a relatively small and stable nucleus of professionals, and patients are referred to the whole team for care. When they talk of the intrinsic aim, they mean the relief of suffering due to physical or mental illness, with the extrinsic aim being the relief of psychological, social and spiritual distress (Randall and Downie 1996, p. 38). The work of Randall and Downie highlights an important tension in how the team is defined in specialist palliative care. Much emphasis is placed today on the centrality of the patient in the planning of treatment and care. Rather than being a passive recipient, many more patients now wish to participate more actively in decision making and establishing a partnership with the health professionals involved (see Chapter 4 of this volume). Many patients will have a broad understanding of the membership of the team and will wish to draw on a wide range of skill and expertise to solve problems as they arise. As Randall and Downie recognize 'From the patient's perspective, the team comprises all those involved in their care' (p. 47), but how do these people come to be involved in the care of the patient? They suggest that the doctors and nurses are present as the core or intrinsic team and others should only be involved at the express request of the patient since they are part of an extrinsic team. In this way, it is felt the autonomy of the patient can be protected as the patient's consent should be sought before any other professional is introduced. Patients, however, need to make informed choices, and the non-medical resources available need to be made known to the patient in such a way as to overcome the dismissal of a resource because of a stereotypical view of the role being described.

The tension regarding definitions of the specialist palliative care team membership and the role of the medical staff has been commented on by Kearney who cautioned against an overemphasis on 'symptomatology' which arose from the attractiveness of separating out the treatment of symptoms from other aspects of care for the person (Kearney 1992). This tendency is contrary to the approach developed by the late Cicely Saunders when she proposed her 'total pain' model (Saunders 1967) and emphasized the importance of an integrated and holistic approach to the patient and the symptoms which the patient presented. Her model highlighted the fact that the experience of pain reported by the patient may have a variety of factors exacerbating the experience in addition to any underlying physical cause. Saunders saw pain as a key which could unlock other problems and requiring multiple interventions before it may be resolved. This led her to formulate a model which included physical, psychological, social, emotional and spiritual components, but as Clark (1999) indicates the model creates its own paradox. Freeing the patient from physical pain can open up other problems of a spiritual, emotional or social nature which may have been hidden or suppressed while the physical pain dominated. These problem areas may then require further discernment and treatment if the patient is ever to become truly pain free. Clark sees that this approach can become an extension of the medical dominion '"There is nothing more we can do" has become "we must think of new possibilities of doing everything". So in resisting one form of disciplinary power (the dominant discourse of bio-medicine) there is a risk of creating another' (p. 734). Clark's review of the concept of 'total pain' leads us to recognize that, if the medical team extend their role to encompass responding to the many factors associated with the experience of pain, then this could be to the exclusion of other health care staff who might have greater experience and skill at addressing the non-physical components. This does not mean that the medical team should not be caring and compassionate and able to discern when other factors may be coming into play—the utilization of *agape* in the writing of Randall and Downie (1996). Nor does it mean that they should not cross disciplinary 'boundaries' since the patient and family frequently choose who they will reveal their concerns to irrespective of the skill of that person to respond to the need. It does mean, however, that whatever discipline a staff member belongs to, that person should be aware of the limits to their ability to meet the needs of every patient and should be willing to seek help or refer to another team member/colleague.

It can be seen that who should or should not be seen as a member of the interdisciplinary team within specialist palliative care is a matter for ongoing debate. A specialist palliative care in-patient unit will be staffed by a variety of disciplines including doctors, nurses, physio- and occupational therapists, social worker and chaplain. Other disciplines may also be employed on a full- or part-time basis or may be invited in according to need. There is then a core multidisciplinary group which may be supplemented by others at various times. Over time, this core group will begin to form itself into an interdisciplinary team, as described by Payne in Chapter 8 of this volume on team building. This is reflected clearly in the guidelines developed by the Scottish Partnership for Palliative Care (1999):

Palliative care is concerned with the whole person—a person's body, mind, emotions, social and family context and spiritual values. The interplay among all the components of the human condition is fully recognised in palliative care. It follows that the provision of palliative care, in order to meet the interrelated needs of the whole person, must itself be inter-related in its practice. Professional people with knowledge and skills ranging from medicine and nursing, the psycho-social and the spiritual, must act as a team with good communication and full co-ordination throughout. Each will know the function of their own skills. Each should understand the limitations of their own skills. Each should recognise the functions and potential of the skills of others [4.1.2].

If the team is to model specialist palliative care, with a holistic approach, it will need to contain a wider mix than just medical and nursing staff. Rather than splitting the membership and task into intrinsic and extrinsic, it may be more helpful to think in terms of certain members or disciplines being more actively involved at various points in the patient's journey. At the time of admission, a patient's primary need may be to have their distressing physical symptoms assessed and, if possible, alleviated. It would not be appropriate to try and assess all the other parameters of care at that point unless the patient clearly raised these as a priority. However, the needs of the family may be very different at this point and they may value having time with a counsellor, chaplain, social worker or psychologist to address some of their anxieties and concerns while the patient's physical needs are being attended to. The role of each of these within the team should not be understood in a narrow way but allow for a degree of overlap because of the developed trust between the post holders. Thus the chaplain may perceive his/her role as wider than providing for religious need and see that there is a need to support the patient in exploring wider existential issues, even if very divergent from those held by the chaplain. Similarly, the social worker may be a very skilled caseworker as well as skilful in steering a course through the benefits regulations. The physiotherapist, in addition to treating the lymphoedema or breathlessness, may also be a good listener to the concerns and anxieties of the patient and able to ease some of them or introduce another team member who can. The availability of other team members to attend to these issues not only would free up the clinical staff to focus on the clinical need but would also ensure that the family felt heard and cared for. The contact with the family may also enable the wider team to become aware of concerns held by the patient and known to the family which could be addressed at a later time.

Within a well-functioning interdisciplinary team, there should be a good degree of trust, respect and confidence in each other's skill and ability. Introducing the patient and family to the team model of working, from the initial contact with any team member, should ensure that the patient is more ready to accept and work with whichever member of the team they meet. This does not mean that team members can assume the patient's readiness to comply with any proffered intervention and, in keeping with good practice, consent should always be obtained by any team member before any form of assessment or intervention is undertaken. This means that the individual team member may initially need to explain their role and what they have to contribute to the care of the patient and why it is thought helpful to be offering the skills of this particular team member. In this way, there will be a closer match to Randall and Downie's observation that patients frequently see themselves drawing on a pool of professionals with whom they can work flexibly and imaginatively to solve problems (p. 47). The core or intrinsic team needs, therefore, to be wider than medical and nursing staff alone. The patient and family need to know what resources are available within the team and how any clinical and personal information shared will be handled within the team, if they are to be able to work flexibly and imaginatively with the pool of professionals (see Chapters 11 and 12 of this volume on ethics and law).

As the patient spends more time in the in-patient unit, he/she will meet with a variety of other people with different roles, such as domestic staff, volunteers, therapists, such as art or music, counsellors, psychiatric services, complementary therapists—aromatherapy or hypnotherapy, and a range of maintenance or ground staff who may relate to the patient in a variety of ways. The level of interaction and involvement of these people with the patient will vary from none at all to a daily interaction with, say, the music therapist through whom the patient may be able to express some of the feelings and reactions they are unable to express verbally or more directly. What is of vital importance is that whoever has encounters with the patient or family should recognize that they are part of the wider network of the in-patient team and should have ways of communicating back to the interdisciplinary team any significant information that may be pertinent to the patient's treatment and care. This implies two things: a degree of insight and training for other staff within the in-patient unit; and recognition of the need to obtain the permission of the patient to share any significant events with the team. Usually patients will give permission if the other person explains why the information may be relevant to their care.

## Volunteers

Volunteers can make an important contribution to the work of the team. Their main goal is to help the professional staff with the enhancement of the patient's quality of life. They bridge the in-patient community with the outside world and often are drawn from the same community as the patient and so may have local knowledge and contacts in common. This can be a benefit or a problem in that patients may welcome talking about people and places known to them, but it can also be upsetting if it evokes unhappy or painful memories from the past or highlights a future hope that is being lost.

Volunteers, as well as assisting in physical care, may have an involvement in social activities within the unit or by taking some patients out into the community for a range of activities. Others may be involved with providing support to patients and families at home. Volunteers need to be carefully selected, trained and supported if they are to be able to sustain their role, because the emotional load may, at times, become hard to bear. This is especially true in those in-patient units which rely heavily on volunteers to participate in bereavement support. Field *et al.* (2004) have shown that the bereavement service in many UK in-patient units is primarily run and staffed by volunteers. Many of the volunteers have themselves been bereaved and offer their services to the hospice as an expression of gratitude for help they themselves received. In itself, this may not be a bad thing, but it does require careful attention to selection, training and support if the volunteers themselves are not to become 'casualties' or drop out of the service. Thinking of team membership, there needs to be a clear link between the work undertaken by the volunteers and the ongoing life of the interdisciplinary team. This might be through an identified individual having responsibility for liaising with the volunteers so that there is a proper degree of 'ownership' of the work they undertake within the unit.

So far, we have focused on the in-patient specialist palliative care unit. The membership of an interdisciplinary team may be very different in other settings and relate to the perceived importance of the service by others, the financial resources available and the ability to recruit key personnel. In other parts of the world, for example, the role of the volunteers may be such that they become the primary carers with support from specialist palliative care workers as illustrated in Box 2.2.

While the example from South India in Box 2.2 may seem distant from the experience of those in better resourced settings, it does show the need for caution when defining who should, or should not, be a member of the team. There are many places where those offering a palliative care service have to cover an extensive geographical area and have limited opportunity or time to meet, share and support other colleagues. In Guyana, for example, there are two palliative care nurses, with a car, seeking to develop a service across an area

---

**Box 2.2** A NEIGHBOURHOOD NETWORK IN KERALA

---

One example of such a programme is that developed in Kerala, South India. The palliative care unit in Calicut started a home care service in 1996 as an extension of the hospital-based palliative care unit. They found that many of their patients in this south Indian state are unable to attend the hospital more than once. Few patients attended for review because they were too ill, had no access to public transport or were too poor to afford to travel. Initially the team tried to encourage relatives to attend and report symptoms and the progress of the patient. However, they soon found that many relatives also failed to attend. The team also wished to empower the patient and family to care for themselves with back up from the centre at Calicut. Medical and nursing resources are limited and so a member of the medical staff visited families in the community, accompanied by trained volunteers. The main selection criteria for volunteers are that they should be compassionate people willing to treat others as equals and able to respect the traditions and values of the other person. There is a large area to cover with many patients, and so it is divided into geographical zones each being covered on a different day. During a visit, there is an assessment of the patient's physical, emotional and socio-economic needs with adjustment to treatment as required. A key aspect of this programme is that the family and patient are taught how to self-care and to involve other family members. This sometimes requires helping the family to resolve disputes between family members so that they can work together. One side effect of this is that families are also beginning to care for sick members of neighbouring families and to share their skills with others. Weekly team meetings are held in Calicut to enable review of difficult problems and any issues arising for team members themselves related to the visits and the nature of the work. In spite of the difficulties created by poverty, transport, state of the roads, lack of telephones, etc., in recent years this work has extended so that there is now an extensive network of volunteers supporting large numbers of families who care for family members with cancer in the community. Imaginative ways of raising funds have also emerged, with local buses and shops contributing 1 rupee per day to the palliative care programme. While miniscule in Western medical terms, these small sums have enabled the service to develop and offer care to large numbers of people who might otherwise have experienced great suffering in their last days.

Account drawn from personal communications with staff involved in the Kerala programme.

See also Neighbourhood Network at

www.painandpalliativecare.org/nnpc/moreinfo.htm

---

of thousands of square miles. The ideal and the possible may be two different things and there is a need for caution in advocating *one* model for teamwork. People who carry the palliative care philosophy and approach to a whole variety of places will need to look at what is possible, even as an interim stage. As others become more aware of the benefits of good palliative care, often especially at government level, then more resources may become available which will allow for more choice in the style of working. Ultimately a point should be reached when the World Health Organization goal of 'achieving the best quality of life for patients and families' is met through a team of professionals working together harmoniously and effectively to deliver the care required.

Within the UK, the person with overall responsibility for the patient's health needs is the family doctor and the primary care team. If the patient is cared for at home, the general practitioner (GP) will provide or coordinate the care and involve palliative care specialists as required. The patient may spend time in the hospital or hospice setting for specific interventions, but will usually return home to the care of the primary care team. If the in-patient unit has a home care team, then specialist palliative care may continue in liaison with the family doctor, and the patient may attend a day unit for reassessment or additional support. Teamwork in palliative care is complex. As in all health care, the GP is the patient's doctor. Normally, in the provision of palliative care at home, the GP will involve others in the team as necessary. Different team members will have greater involvement at various times. Specialists with particular skills may join the team briefly, or for specific purposes, and volunteers can provide support and companionship to complement the professional input. Whether or not they are seen as part of the core team, it is essential that their contribution is valued and there exists a mechanism to enable good communication between the core team and those with a more peripheral relationship with the patient and family. The way in which the setting in which care is provided can affect communication and development of team working will be discussed in Chapter 3 of this volume.

## Conclusion

Within the common understanding of specialist palliative care, it is expected that care will be delivered through the work of a well-coordinated team rather than through a group of people only loosely interconnected. It is too easy to fall through the 'holes' in a group. Groups are an important part of our work and personal life and, while the terms group and team may be used interchangeably by some writers, it is believed here that the team concept is different and more appropriate to palliative care. The smaller size, the high degree of mutual accountability and focus on the task with flexibility of leadership all contribute to a greater chance of attaining well-coordinated quality care.

It is the patient himself or herself, together with spouse, family or close friends, who remains the central focus throughout. From the time of diagnosis until the time of discharge or death, the patient and family will encounter a wide range of people who will contribute to their treatment and care. The diagnosis will usually be confirmed following investigations within an acute hospital setting. Primarily this will involve a medical doctor who will review the results and discuss them with the patient and professional colleagues. These professional colleagues will include other medical staff, nurse specialists, pathologist, oncologist, and maybe a counsellor and/or chaplain.

To avoid confusion and irritation by having to rehearse their story many times, patients will expect there to be good communication between team members who may be working in a range of different settings. This is a prerequisite for continuity of care and is in keeping with generally accepted understanding of the aims of palliative care and reflected in the NICE (UK) guidance for supportive care. In line with this guidance, it is important that the needs of the patient are assessed and reassessed at various points along the care pathway, beginning at the time of diagnosis. Who the key people are in assessing and meeting those needs will depend on what the patient is experiencing and the setting within which they find themselves. If they fail to work effectively with each other, it will be the patient and family who will lose out.

It is by continuing to focus on the patient that any team, however wide ranging in skills or settings, will be able to ensure the quality of life and continuity of care which are the twin objectives of palliative care.

## References

Belbin RM (2000). *Beyond the Team*. Butterworth-Heinemann, Oxford, p. 15.

Cane S (1996). *Kaizen Strategies for Winning Through People*. Pitman Publishing, London, p. 116.

Clark D (1999). 'Total pain', disciplinary power and the body in the work of Cicely Saunders, 1958–1967. *Social Science and Medicine* **49**, 727–736.

Cummings I (1998). The interdisciplinary team. In: Doyle D, Hanks GWC and MacDonald N, ed. *Oxford Textbook of Palliative Medicine*, 2nd edn. Oxford University Press, Oxford.

Field D, Reid D, Payne S and Relf M. (2004). Survey of UK hospice and specialist palliative care adult bereavement services. *International Journal of Palliative Nursing* **10**, 569–576.

Harré R and Lamb R (eds) (1986). *The Dictionary of Personality and Social Psychology*. Blackwell, Oxford.

Holpp L (1997). Teams: it's all in the planning. *Training and Development* **51**, 44–47.

Kearney M (1992). Palliative medicine—just another specialty. *Palliative Medicine* **6**, 39–46.

Kravitz DA and Martin B (1986). Ringelmann rediscovered: the original article. *Journal of Personality and Social Psychology* May, 936–941.

NICE (2004). *Guidance on Cancer Services: Improving Supportive and Palliative Care for Adults with Cancer*. National Institute for Clinical Excellence, London.

Randall F and Downie RS (1996). *Palliative Care Ethics: A Good Companion*. Oxford University Press, Oxford.

Saunders C (1967). *The Management of Terminal Illness*. Hospital Medicine Publications, London.

Schein E (1988). *Organizational Psychology*, 3rd edn. Prentice Hall, Harlow, UK.

Scottish Partnership for Palliative Care (1999) Section 4.1.2 www.palliativecarescotland. org.uk

Sherif M and Sherif CW (1969). *Social Psychology*. Harper & Row, New York.

World Health Organization (2002). *National Cancer Control Programmes: Policies and Guidelines*. WHO, Geneva.

# 3

# The effect of the setting on the work of the team

*Michaela Bercovitch and Abraham Adunsky*

One of the main issues in palliative medicine is cooperation between patients, families and health professionals. When we were invited to discuss the effect of the setting on the work of the team in palliative medicine, we were both amazed to realize that this controversial subject has hardly been researched. We came to the conclusion that the process of care has not been as widely studied as the quality of care.

Having been members of a palliative care team for >15 years, we thought that nothing could be simpler than writing about team work. This is a well-known area for both of us—as part of a team and as teachers about team work—so we thought there would be no problem in finding relevant literature and worldwide examples of different models of team work in order to describe various ways of communication and collaboration between team members in a variety of settings.

As we both live in a very small country, distances are not a major impediment for teams to meet and coordinate their work. We were not aware of the problems of loneliness experienced by some team members in other parts of the world because of their greater distances or lack of organized services.

We also became aware of the paucity of literature in this particular domain. Whilst many research projects were performed in rural areas concerning the quality of care, very little has been published about the process and problems of team work in various settings.

So, after a long period of thinking and searching, we decided to begin this chapter with a description of the interactive work of a team comprised of various health professionals, and then to apply this to palliative care by using examples from various studies.

During the last century, a dramatic epidemiological change has occurred: life expectancy has increased and people are older when they, die but, at the same time, the incidence of chronic diseases has increased. More and more people die as a result of serious chronic disease, suffering from multiorgan failure towards the end of life (Davies and Higginson 2004). Palliative care patients have a variety of complex physical, psycho-social and spiritual needs which cannot be met and resolved by a single individual (Jeffrey 2004). Towards the end of life, sick people need to be in familiar surroundings, together with family and friends, they feel the need to be involved in the decision-making process regarding their own treatment and they need to communicate honestly with their caregivers. All these are paramount requirements of the palliative caring process.

In the last 50 years, we have witnessed the explosive development of palliative medicine and the hospice concept which are designed to meet the needs and expectations of terminally ill patients and their families. It seems that this is the best way to care for them at the end of life.

The concept of 'relief of total pain' introduced by Dame Cicely Saunders, is reflected in the most recent definition of palliative care:

Palliative care consists of an approach that improves the quality of life of patients and their families facing the problems associated with life threatening illness, through the prevention and relief of suffering by means of early identification and impeccable assessment and treatment of pain and other problems—physical, psycho-social and spiritual (World Health Organizaton 2002).

This definition of palliative care expresses the necessity for a 'partnership between a team of different health professionals and a client in a participatory, collaborative and well coordinated approach to shared decision making around health issues' (Orchard and Curran 2003). Introducing the patient and the family as active members of the team compels them to assume responsibility for his/her health, changing the balance in the decision-making process (Orchard *et al.* 2005; Chapter 4 of this volume).

Services are provided by patient-centred and clinically directed interdisciplinary teams of patients, their families, and health care professionals and volunteers. These teams have a high capacity for assessment, drawing up a list of problems, offering other options and selecting the best alternative, thus creating a treatment plan, the last step being the application of the treatment, under the direct supervision of the team members. Most important in maintaining a healthy and productive team are mutual trust, free-flowing communication between members, strong collaboration, respect of each other and recognition and resolution of unexpected conflicts. Conflict within teams remains one of the most important barriers to team survival. It may reflect problems between members of the team as a result of ignorance of the values of practice of other disciplines, poor communication, overappreciation of one discipline, overlapping competencies and responsibilities, and even chauvinism. (Mariano 1998; Chapter 7 of this volume). Another source of conflict may be the different points of view, rules or expectations of a larger system within which the team operates. Rigid bureaucratic old systems which are not compatible with the strongly built relationship and principles of work within an interdisciplinary team may cause high staff turnover and rotation of health professionals (Drinka 1994). In today's new health system, it seems to be more efficient to achieve goals through cooperation rather than through powerful competition (Forbes and Fitzsimons 1993). Another critical problem within interdisciplinary teams might be the building of leadership: who will be the main manager? In traditional teams, the manager was and still is the physician. In interdisciplinary teams, the role of the leader should be flexible and dependent on the unique patient situation. Leadership should not be a manifestation of hierarchy but of excellence in clinical problem solving (Crawford and Price 2003).

Even if interdisciplinary work proves itself and improvement of the organizational effectiveness is obvious, there are some barriers that may have a negative effect on the smooth working of the whole team. These barriers could be the different settings in which the teams works, very wide geographical areas, poor funding or differences of opinion between members of the palliative care team and the general practitioners (GPs). A lack of understanding of the pressures experienced by people because of the setting in which they work might also lead to lack of prioritizing of team meetings and collaboration between members of the team, lack of agreement as to the concept of total collaboration and different forms of organization.

The classically recognized interdisciplinary team incorporates specialized professionals and paraprofessionals working together to achieve the same final goal: the best quality of life in the time remaining for patient and his/her close family and friends. Because of the complexity of this goal, a team has to comprise:

- The patient's attending physician
- Palliative care specialized physicians
- Specialized palliative care registered nurses
- Social workers trained in working with the terminally ill and their families
- Chaplains or spiritual counsellors
- Trained volunteers
- Hospice aid workers with palliative education and clinical experience
- Bereavement counsellors
- The occasional help of other professionals such as a psychiatrist, orthopaedist, etc., might be required.

These teams are geared to work in harmony and to provide excellent interdisciplinary hospice care. However, this can be affected by the setting in which the team operates.

## One place centralized team

The traditional, well-organized interdisciplinary team is concentrated in one place; each member has his own area of care but the information is shared in team meetings once a week. In these meetings, all the disciplines participate, as this is the place for elaboration of the treatment plan. Depending on the case, some of the disciplines might have a higher impact on the success of the treatment than others. *Flowing and continuous communication* between the team members is even more important when the patient's general condition deteriorates. Moreover, telling the truth, and keeping an open attitude have to be at the base of every interdisciplinary palliative care team.

Creating and maintaining an effective interdisciplinary palliative care team, even when localized in the same place, is not an easy process. Working in an interdisciplinary team is difficult and different from the classic multidisciplinary teams where the representatives of each medical discipline work independently. The treatment is determined by the physician in charge, while the patient and the patient's family have very limited say in the therapeutic decisions. In an interdisciplinary palliative team, the professional boundaries are less important, the leadership being dependent on the task at hand and not on professional hierarchy (Council of Europe 2003). Secondly, interdisciplinary teams include non-professionals (volunteers, patients and family members) (Cummings 1998) as direct participants in the team decision-making process. Thirdly, because of the complexity of problems to be assessed and dealt with, communication between members of the team is one of the most important facets of the teamwork. Fourthly, conflicting issues, role ambiguity and overlapping may negatively influence the team's capacity to achieve its goals (Crawford and Price 2003).

Therefore, in order to build a viable team, some selection criteria for team members is necessary. Flexibility, ability to support colleagues, respect for others and awareness of what is meant by trust are the most important qualities required for a future team member (West 1993).

Once the team is formed, coordination of the work and the maintenance of a 'healthy team' have to be the main purpose of the leaders. Again, the importance of communication between team members should be stressed. Allowing enough time for periodic discussions of common goals, discussing individual roles and problems and supporting each other are the basic tasks to attend to, in order to achieve job satisfaction for the whole team. The setting in which the team operates in relation to other service providers (where such exist) can be very influential in determining the effectiveness of their worth.

A specialized team has to organize itself around a common programme. In an in-patient palliative hospice unit, the ward rounds have high priority. Working together means meeting with all the team members before beginning the round and pinpointing the most difficult problems. Usually during rounds the physician acts as the leader while nurses and social workers act as patient advocates. After rounds, it is usual to discuss the treatment plans with those patients who are able to participate and their families.

The situation is different in home visits where the nurse usually sees the patient alone. This visit should be thoroughly prepared. The team should create a list of problems related to the patient and suggest an appropriate course of action to solve them. A full report of the visit is vital for all members of the team. The report should be in writing and completed at the weekly meetings. The meetings should be the main occasion for discussing the problems, planning future intervention and deciding on the action of each discipline in its area of specialty. Even in those cases where the care is delivered far away from the team base, it should be coordinated with the work undertaken by the rest of the team to ensure continuity of care between in-patient, day care and home care.

During the weekly meetings, success and failure of the programme should be discussed and associated lessons learned. Mutual respect for the competence and role of each team member is vital.

The following is an example of negative behaviour by a team leader within an in-patient unit, which in part was related to interpretation of role within an hierarchical setting.

In one of the regular team meetings, a controversial problem was discussed.

One of the hospice patients suffered a massive haemorrhagic episode caused by the dislodgement of a nephrostome. After consulting with the ward nurse and the physician who were on duty during the night and, after talking to the family, it was decided to perform a blood transfusion. In the morning, the medical director strongly disagreed with the decision and made this very clear to everyone on the ward. In his opinion, the correct therapeutic approach should have been to consider sedation and to persuade the family members to accept it. This attitude caused a lot of confusion among the team members, and when the problem was again discussed during the weekly meeting the team leader tried to impose his point of view without considering any counter-arguments. Using high tones, he made some critical comments about the competence of the other physician and left the room, leaving everybody embarrassed. This unsolved conflict caused confusion and created a negative atmosphere which lasted for a long time. Such lack of communication and ineffective leadership may lead to distrust and demoralization amongst team members. The use of a higher position on the administrative ladder to force a line of treatment, while denying other team members or the patient's family the right to participate in the therapeutic decision, is against the very essence of the interdisciplinary team concept.

The above example illustrates the confusion between the administrative position of the team member and his caregiver function within the interdisciplinary team. A nurse in an administrative position who is the caregiver for a small number of patients, as a member of the managerial staff, is also responsible for all the patients on the ward and for the work of all the other nurses and may try to exert her authority. This might cause real trouble in the team. The other nurses might feel hurt because their autonomy was curtailed. This is, in fact, a leadership conflict between the administrative manager and the caregiver who is temporally managing the case at the clinical level. This kind of behaviour is mostly encountered in large settings with rigid organizational rules and a culture which reinforces hierarchical patterns of work.

The interdisciplinary team must be considered as an independent forum. Interference of outsiders in the management of the team or in the clinical process must be filtered by the team manager, otherwise the outcome might be destructive to the functioning of the team and quality of care to the patient.

It is the role of the team manager to protect the team autonomy. When conflicting loyalty leans toward a powerful administrative position, not only the team but also the entire programme will suffer even to the extent that survival of the programme might be in danger When the team manager is more oriented towards the administrative aspect, and the interplay of his/her conflicting functions is not well assimilated, the flexibility in roles is jeopardized and the interdisciplinary teamwork concept is trampled (see Chapter 5 of this volume)

In some settings, in-patient and out-patient hospices are combined, but because of funding issues and organizational constraints their administrative affiliation might be different. For example, the in-patient unit might be funded by a large medical centre, whilst the home care team is controlled by a private society or a charity. In spite of this, both teams should work together in perfect coordination, helping patients from the community to be admitted to the in-patient unit, or vice versa. If, however, because of the bureaucracy, the teams work independently and never meet to discuss special cases, communication between the teams will remain at the minimal level of 'transferring the case' from one venue to the other with no continuity of care. Although sharing the same goals, the two teams are almost disconnected. Even worse, the two management systems may have different visions about what palliative care is and does.

Continuity of care is one of the most important factors in the last phase of life and should be easier to achieve in a centralized team. If continuity of care is disrupted, it might affect the whole system of care ('the capacity to live and develop') and thus endanger the whole palliative care program (*Webster's New Collegiate Dictionary* 1995; NICE 2004).

## Rural and remote settings?

We analysed several problems that can occur when the teams are working in one central place, where all the conditions for good communication and collaboration exist but problems may still arise. However, nowadays, there are millions of people suffering and dying at home in rural areas. Who is responsible for the care of the dying and their families when hospitals or medical centres are too far from their homes? Is it realistic to organize a real interdisciplinary team for each little settlement? Are there enough funding resources? The answer is probably no, even though nowadays all efforts are being made to introduce well-organized home palliative care wherever there is suffering due to life-threatening disease.

There are some conditions which make ideal care for the end of life possible, even in rural areas. The ideal structure may comprise (Kevin *et al.* 2003):

- A GP with some knowledge of palliative care
- A specialized palliative care team
- An in-patient facility nearby, for difficult cases.

This model was tried in Australia with fairly good results. However, there were many impediments affecting the communication between the members of the team:

- The GPs' lack of knowledge and skills in palliative care
- Lack of time to provide appropriate care and to hold team meetings
- Inappropriate remuneration (Reymond *et al.* 2003)
- The preference of GPs to be the main coordinators and to consider other members as assistants in providing physical, emotional and spiritual care (Kevin *et al.* 2003)
- The competing role definitions that stem from the different working cultures of GP and palliative care teams (Mitchel *et al.* 2002).

GPs hold the primary responsibility (within the UK) for the health care needs of people within the community, therefore these barriers have to be resolved in order to achieve good communication between GPs and the other palliative care team members, thus enabling quality of care at home, based on interdisciplinary team work. Lack of communication and collaboration between GPs and other professionals may generate conflict between health providers and result in numerous disciplines caring independently for the same patient and not functioning as an interdisciplinary team having the same goals and interests.

In some rural areas, the only palliative care provider might be a specialist nurse. In these situations, the rural nurses provide complex services, similar to those often delivered by medical or allied health professionals in large centres. These nurses sometimes establish relationships with their clients and their families beyond the professional context (Rosenberg and Canning 2004).

Community-based specialist nurses often work in geographical and professional isolation that might cause a barrier to professional development and certainly a lack in the services provided. Creatively, they organize the services using as team members and support resources the 'receptionist, the administrator, the police and/or the school' to help in many of their activities (Kovacich 1996). When the resources are not sufficient and there are not enough opportunities to develop a face to face interdisciplinary team, the specialist nurses may seek support from community workers rather than other nursing or health care colleagues. This is mainly because the community worker may be more readily available at the time when support is needed and has a good understanding of the particular problems which the patient and family may be presenting.

Other professionals such as GPs, social workers, psychotherapists and others are used occasionally when needed, but may not always be available to care for terminally ill people at home.

Another solution found in conditions of poorly resourced services or geographically distanced teams was the case manager approach. This means a community-based case management approach, aimed to care for patients at home in the last year of life.

In 1998, a project plan was elaborated by the Mount Sinai School of Medicine, Franklin Health and South Carolina Blue Cross, Blue Shield (Meier *et al.* 2004). By using a local nurse as case coordinator, a remote physician manager and a clinical account manager, Meier *et al.* proposed to establish a service in which the communication and coordination of the treatment between the patient, the palliative care team and the primary physician was maintained by electronic means. The most problematic aspect was collaboration between the nurse and the physician. In an attempt to improve the communication, the case manager sent, by fax, to the physicians a one-page 'Practical Guide to Communication Styles in Clinical Practice'. The project showed that in the beginning the nurses entered the project with some scepticism and insecurity regarding assessments, interventions and communication with others, but at the end they demonstrated an enthusiastic attitude, acted as advocates for their patients and were able to form a real team with the attending physicians. This created a community-based, successful palliative care framework, outside of a formal in-patient hospice programme (Meier *et al.* 2004).

In 1996, Elsey and McIntre, in their study of a similar service structure, concluded in their survey that there existed a lack of supportive collegial communication and personal debriefing (Elsey and McIntre 1996). A further study by McConigley found that the only source of support for rural nurses was within their own families (McConigley *et al.* 2000). More than that, the nurses working in rural and remote areas complained of a lack of access to continuing education and professional development because of a multitude of factors, such as distances, problems with staffing replacement, family problems and costs (McCarthy and Heghey 1999). All these barriers have a negative impact on the delivery of palliative care services in rural settings. In essence, the nurses are working as 'sole practitioners' without teams and without psychological and educational support. This situation has many negative implications on the care of the terminally ill and their families.

In 2003, the Palliative Care Society in Australia published a 'planning guide' designed to offer a solution for most of the difficulties regarding palliative care in Australia in general and in rural and remote settings in particular. The guide accentuates the necessity for teamwork, emphasizes the importance of creating effective communication among professionals and, when the distance constitutes a problem, recommends telephone or video conferencing to maintain the teamwork process (Currow and Nightingale 2003). The guide offers suggestions on how to maintain communication between team members separated by distances and how to provide a strong support system for the whole group by means of networking. There are, of course, some impediments in using computer-mediated communication. These are expensive tools and their use requires good technical knowledge of the computer and good infrastructure such as a reliable power and telephone supply. Nevertheless, the research attests that computer-mediated communication systems, while beneficial, are less effective than face to face group meetings, especially in difficult situations or emergencies when communication and support are required immediately (Hightower and Sayeed 1995).

The clear message resulting from all the above studies is that communication between members of the interdisciplinary team is a must. In 2004, Bakitas *et al.* published in the *Journal of Palliative Medicine* a proposal of a new project aimed at introducing palliative services in different settings (Bakitas *et al.* 2004). The idea was to introduce a palliative care nurse or a nurse practitioner who would coordinate the care of the patients and families across clinical specialties and community agencies. Three different settings were chosen: a tertiary academic centre, a rural location and a private haemato-oncology group.

In the academic centre, this tentative arrangement generated a lot of resistance from the local oncologist and the rest of the oncology team. The palliative professionals were perceived as 'outsiders' to be kept at a distance or as a redundant service interposed between the patient and the local team. In the rural setting, it was very quickly seen that supplementing the services with a skilled hospice social worker was absolutely essential because of the large variety of problems and responsibilities of the nurse. Together these two professionals were able to stabilize communication with other members of the local multidisciplinary team. The introduction and stabilization of palliative care consultation and collaboration was simpler in the setting of the private haemato-oncology group.

This study demonstrates that ignorance regarding the role of palliative care makes it very difficult for individual palliative care professionals to be accepted by the multidisciplinary team whatever the setting, and has training and educational implications (see Chapter 10 of this volume).

## Nursing homes

Another important setting for palliative care are nursing homes, which are significant care providers in the UK, Europe and elsewhere. Some models of beneficial collaboration between nursing homes and local hospices and palliative care institutions are described in the literature (Manson 2003; Touch *et al.* 2003).

Touch *et al.* showed that the assimilation of the palliative care methodology within the nursing home organization was a long and challenging process, involving intensive education of the medical, psycho-social and administrative personnel. On the other hand, the development and introduction of simpler palliative care assessment tools that decreased the burden of the related paperwork made the palliative care approach acceptable to the local teams. The last step was to organize regular scheduled interdisciplinary palliative care team meetings, led by the medical director of the team. These meetings were open to medical personnel and to residents and their families, allowing for the discussion and resolution of both medical and psycho-social issues. The families were also encouraged to be more involved in the decision-making process and in resolving difficult problems.

Although the meetings were held after hours and without pay, the involvement of the physicians increased because of the valuable outcome of these meetings and their effectiveness for the daily work with dying patients. One of the major problems facing the newly created team was the staff turnover. Every time when more than one staff member left, it was necessary to start all over again. Touch *et al.* conclude that in nursing home facilities, it is not necessary to bring in a new team to coordinate the palliative care services for residents. Using the existing teams seems to be just as successful. Bringing the administrators, physicians, nurses, families and residents, social workers and dieticians from the nursing home together in order to discuss and decide on the treatment plan on a weekly basis was the major success factor. Another positive result was the decrease in the number of referrals to the regional hospital because staff felt more able to care for the patients within their nursing home (see also Katz and Peace 2003).

## Out-patient clinics

Another setting in which palliative care may be provided is the out-patient clinic. In their paper, Rabow *et al.* (2003) described the work of palliative care teams in out-patient clinics. The social worker, pharmacist, chaplain, psychologist, clinical artists and physicians constituted the team, and the model of work was a social worker-centred case management approach. In this case, the social worker was the first team member to meet with the patient, take a complete report on physical symptoms and conduct a comprehensive psycho-social assessment. The second step was the presentation of the assessment to the whole team, followed by discussion and recommendations for the primary care physician who remained the primary caregiver. The case discussions were repeated periodically and the palliative care team was involved, as necessary, in the organization of support services for the patient, feedback for the primary care physician or direct consult-ation with the patients and their families (Rabow *et al.* 2003)

However, even if this seems to be an excellent and effective model for continuity of services, its implementation was made difficult by the poor cooperation of the personal physicians who were reluctant to accept the team's clinical recommendations and even unwilling to recommend the pro-gramme to the patients. Other impediments faced by the palliative care team were refusals to participate in the programme because of transportation prob-lems or patient mobility issues. These facts again demonstrate that communi-cation is the most important factor in the proper functioning of palliative care teams. Therefore, it is advisable to invite the primary care physicians to the periodical meetings and, with the palliative care team working within the out-patient's department, encouraging them to be a part of the decision-making process as team members and, at the same time, to be advocates for their patients. Thus the palliative care approach and treatment plan, as a consensus of all the involved caregivers, will be more easily accepted.

Continuity of care is of major importance and the work mode where the palliative care team has only a consultative role might not be sufficient for many patients, nor for their primary care physicians. In these cases, finding the common ground where both the palliative and oncological approaches coordinate to provide effective treatment is essential. Placing an isolated 'specialist' nurse or doctor in a very treatment-curative-focused out-patient setting often creates a range of difficulties. The setting, in which the lone specialist is trying to demonstrate the validity and importance of a differing approach and focus, will certainly influence the effectiveness and quality of their care, and could demoralize a lone worker.

## Palliative mobile teams in the hospital

In some large medical centres, the palliative care approach is promoted by mobile palliative care teams that provide advice, consultation, support and training for relevant hospital departments. The first such team was that estab-lished at St Thomas' Hospital in London (Bates *et al.* 1981) and it became a model for many others which were developed in later years. The European Commission described the experience of such mobile teams during a 4-year period of activity in their project of promoting the development and integration of palliative care mobile support teams in the hospital. The pallia-tive care mobile teams had a multidisciplinary composition, and their direct involvement in the care of the patients was negotiated with the referring teams, which usually retained responsibility for the decision making and provision of the treatment (see European Commission 2004). Usually, these teams consisted of 3–4 members and took direct action regarding the difficult complex cases in the whole institution. Their function was to contact, assess, elaborate the treatment plan and make advisory indications to the primary hospital care teams. The treatment plan was elaborated during periodic team meetings. The team had to take into consideration the organizational and treatment approach distinctions between the various hospital departments (internal departments, surgical, oncological, geriatrics, etc.). The work of such a team is stressful. The study of their activities in large medical centres showed a low level of autonomy due to hospital restrictions that predisposed the team members to conflict with the institutional administration. This stressful environment led to instability in the team's membership and functioning. Another problem mentioned as affecting the good functioning of the team was the advisory character of the team. The departmental medical teams tend to consider their activity as 'giving only indications' and 'leaving' the 'dirty jobs' for others. The result was poor support for the terminally ill and their families. The recommendations of the European commission were to create a strong collaboration and fluid communication with the administrative and managerial staff and different departmental teams through systematic information of the objectives, competencies and functioning mode of these mobile teams.

## Conclusions

Over the years, the interdisciplinary model for palliative care has proved itself as a viable and effective approach for the complex health needs of patients in general and those suffering from life-threatening diseases in particular.

The effectiveness of interdisciplinary teamwork has been analysed in many studies (Saunders 1993; Woodruf 1993; World Health Oranization 1997). Working in a collaborative manner, establishing a partnership between the client and the health care providers may improve the quality of care, client satisfaction and the cost-effectiveness of the services.

However, as we have demonstrated, there are many obstacles in the way to achievement of the interdisciplinary team goals:

- Organizational structuralism (Karackhardt 1990; Gummer 1994; Adams *et al.* 1998)
- Power relationships between health care professionals (Vrfenderburgh and Bender 1994; Blair and Buessler 1998)
- Power relationships between health care professionals and their clients (Decker 1997; Sitzia and Wood 1997.

In this chapter, we have looked into the variety of challenges faced by the palliative care team imposed by the different settings in which they function. We also learned about mitigation plans and other team efforts to enable the programme to survive and to continue to provide high quality care for patients and their families. After 30 years of practising palliative medicine in general and within interdisciplinary teams in particular, we can state that the complete integration of this discipline into the health care system has not yet been accomplished.

Various electronic means such as computer-mediated communication through networking and video conferencing as a means of support for the isolated practitioner or team on the one hand, and intensive education for the members of the multidisciplinary team and the administrative personnel in large medical centres on the other, are some of the tools of this struggle.

In spite of all the issues and difficulties mentioned, the people involved in this kind of practice described their work as 'a way of life' (Webster and Krisjanson 2002). The work of palliative care brought together the simple recognition of the individual's value, encouraged personal growth and offered the possibility to be a part of a vibrant environment. Their services, felt and valued across various settings and communities, offer a unique way of preserving the dignity and self-respect of the terminally ill person facing imminent death.

## References

Adams A, Bond S and Hale CA (1998). Nursing organizational practice and its relationship with other features of ward organization and job satisfaction. *Journal of Advanced Nursing* 27, 1212–1222.

Bakitas M, Stevens M, Ahles T, Kirn M, Skalla K, Kane N and Greenberg ER, The Project Enable Co-Investigators (2004). Project ENABLE: a palliative care demonstration: project for advanced care patients in three settings. *Journal of Palliative Medicine* 7, 363–372.

Bates T, Hoy A, Clarke D and Laird P (1981). A new concept of hospice care: St Thomas' terminal care support team. *Lancet* 1, 1201–1203.

Blair JD and Buessler JA (1998). Competitive forces in the medical group industry: a stakeholder perspective. *Health Care Management Review* 23, 7–27.

Council of Europe (2003). *Recommendation [Rec 2003] of the Committee of Ministers to Member States on the Organization of Palliative Care.* Council of Europe, pp. 64–68.

Crawford BG and Price DS (2003). Team working: palliative care as a model of interdisciplinary practice. *Medical Journal of Australia* 179 (Suppl), 32–34.

Cummings I. (1998). The interdisciplinary team. In: Doyle D, Hanks GWC and MacDonald N, ed. *Oxford Textbook of Palliative Medicine*, 2nd edn. Oxford University Press, Oxford, pp. 19–30.

Currow CD and Nightingale ME (2003). 'A Planning Guide': developing a consensus document for palliative care services provision. *Medical Journal of Australia* **179** (Suppl), 523–525.

Davies E and Higginson IJ (eds) (2004). *Palliative Care—The Solid Facts*. WHO, Geneva, pp. 8–10.

Decker FM (1997). Occupational and non-occupational factors in job satisfaction and psychological distress among nurses. *Research in Nursing and Health* **20**, 453–464.

Drinka TYK (1994). Interdisciplinary geriatric teams: approaches to conflict as an indicator potential to model teamwork. *Educational Gerontology* **20**, 87–103.

Elsey B and McIntre J (1996). Assessing a support and learning network for palliative care workers in a country area of South Australia. *Australian Journal of Rural Health* **4**, 159–164.

European Commission (2004). *Quality of Life and Management of Living Resources*. The fifth framework program 1998–2002. Result of the European project collaboration funded by the European Commission.

Forbes EJ and Fitzsimons V (1993). Education: the key for holistic interdisciplinary collaboration. *Holistic Nursing Practice* **7**, 1–10.

Gummer B (1994). Getting and staying in the loop: networking and organizational power. *Administration in Social Work* **18**, 107–123.

Hightower RT and Sayeed L (1995). The impact of computer mediated communication systems on biased group discussion. *Computers in Human Behavior* **11**, 33–44.

Jeffrey D (2004).Communication with professionals. In: Doyle D, Hanks GFK, Cherny N and Calman K, ed. *Oxford Textbook of Palliative Medicine*, 3rd edn. Oxford University Press, Oxford, pp. 107–12.

Karackhardt D (1990). Assessing the political landscape: structure, cognition and power in organizations. *Administrative Science Quarterly* **35**, 342–369.

Katz JS and Peace S (2003). *End of Life in Care Homes: A Palliative Care Approach*. Oxford University Press, Oxford.

Kevin JY, Behrndt MM, Christofer J and Mitchel GK (2003). Palliative care at home: general practitioners working with palliative care teams. *Medical Journal of Australia* **179** (Suppl), 38–40.

Kovacich J (1996). Interdisciplinary team turning on the information superhighway. *Journal of Interprofessional Care* **10**, 111–119.

Manson LC (2003). Creating excellent palliative care in nursing homes. *Journal of Palliative Medicine* **6**, 7–9.

Mariano C (1998). The case for interdisciplinary collaboration. *Nursing Outlook* **37**, 285–288.

McCarthy A and Heghey D. (1999). Rural nursing in Australian context. In: Aranda S, O'Connor, ed. *Palliative Care*. AustMed, Ascot Vale, Australia, pp. 83–101.

McConigley R, Kristjanson L and Morgan A (2000). Palliative care nursing in rural Western Australia. *International Journal of Palliative Nursing* **6**, 80–90.

Meier D, Thar W, Jordan A, Goldhirsh LS, Sin A and Morrison RJ (2004). Integrating case management and palliative care. *Journal of Palliative Medicine* **7**, 119–133.

Mitchel GK, De Jong IC, Del Mar CB, Clavarino AM and Kennedy R (2002). General practitioner attitudes to conferences: how can we increase participation and effectiveness? Editorial. *Medical Journal of Australia*, **177**, 95–97.

NICE (2004). *Guidance on Cancer Services: Improving Supportive and Palliative Care for Adults with Cancer*. National Institute for Clinical Excellence, London.

Orchard CA, Curran V and Kabene S (2005). Creating a culture for interdisciplinary collaborative professional practice. *Medical Education online* (www.med-ed-online.org) 1–13.

Orchard CA and Curran V (2003). *Centres of Excellence for Interdisciplinary Collaborative Professional Practice*. Prepared for the Office of Nursing Policy: Health Canada, Government of Canada.

Rabow WM, Petersen J, Schanche K, Dibble LS and McPhee JS (2003). The comprehensive care team: a description of a controlled trial of care at the beginning of the end of life. *Journal of Palliative Medicine* 6, 489–499.

Reymond E, Mitchel G, McGrath B and Welch D (2003). *Research into the Educational Training and Support Needs of General Practitioners in Palliative Care*. Report to the Department of Health and Aging, Brisbane, Mt Olivet Health Services (Executive summary available at www.mtolivet.org.au\research\research%20projects\research_project.htm)

Rosenberg PJ and Canning FD (2004). Palliative care by nurses in rural and remote practice. *Australian Journal of Rural Health* 12, 166–171.

Saunders C (1993). Foreword. In: Doyle D, Hanks GWC and MacDonald N, ed. *Oxford Textbook of Palliative Medicine*. Oxford University Press, Oxford, pp. v–vii.

Sitzia J and Wood N (1997). Patient satisfaction: a review of issues and concepts. *Social Science and Medicine* 45, 1829–1843.

Touch H, Parish P and Romer LA (2003). Integrating palliative care into nursing homes. *Journal of Palliative Medicine* 6, 297–309.

Vrfenderburgh D and Bender Y (1994). The hierarchical abuse of power in work organizations. *Journal of Business Ethics* 17, 1337–1347.

Webster J and Krisjanson JL (2002) 'But isn't it depressing?' 'The vitality' of palliative care. *Journal of Palliative Care* 18, 15–24.

*Webster's New Collegiate Dictionary* (1995). Thomas Allen & Son, Ontario, p. 1309.

West T (1993). The work of the interdisciplinary team. In: Saunders C and Sykes N, ed. *The Management of Terminal Malignant Disease*, 3rd edn. Edward Arnold, London, pp. 226–235.

World Health Organization (1997). *The World Health Report*. WHO, Geneva.

World Health Organization (2002). *National Cancer Control Programs: Policies and Managerial Guidelines*, 2nd edn. WHO, Geneva

Woodruf R (1993). *Palliative Medicine: Symptomatic and Supportive Care for Patients with Advanced Cancer and AIDS*, 2nd edn. Asperula, Victoria, Australia, pp. 3–25

# 4

# User involvement—the patient and carer as team members?

*David Oliviere*

The patient should preside over his/her own dying

Lamerton (1986)

'Interdisciplinary teams will form, and reform and change like patterns in a kaleidoscope in the changing scenarios in the health care systems—but what unifies the whole enterprise is the patient whose story is the common thread' (Lickiss *et al.* 2004). The patient and carer are not totally helpless entities to be ministered to by the multiprofessional team (Small 2005). That palliative care be person-centred, with patients and carers retaining as much choice and control as possible, is one of the sacred tenets of the work and of high priority for professionals (Clark 2005). User involvement recognizes the potential contribution a patient and carer can make to the process and outcome of palliative care—after all, whose illness, care and death is it anyway? At all levels of care, user involvement is consistent with treating patients and carers as whole people, and reflected in the UK Government's 'Expert Patient Programme' (NHS 2006).

Lickiss *et al.* remind us that throughout the illness, the patient will have contact with many teams, for differing lengths of time as he/she passes from general practitioner (GP), oncologist, nurse, social worker, therapist to even a person holding legal status, such as enduring power of attorney (Lickiss *et al.* 2004). An ill person who uses health services and multiprofessional teams is also a person with intelligence, a social life, likely to have had professional and other life skills, endearing and less endearing personality traits and an active cognitive processing of the world. He/she is someone with likes and dislikes and opinions. As the illness progresses, some of these aspects are enveloped by disabling symptoms, appointments and interviews, crises and, increasingly, being on the receiving end of help (Small and Rhodes 2000). Opportunities to give are reduced or disguised. User involvement can tap into the healthy sides of people and affirm the palliative care ethic that a *dying* patient is a *living* person (Oliviere 2001).

User involvement remains a challenge as well as an artform for the multi-professional team whose patients are at the centre of care: how this is achieved, sustained and services enhanced is the subject matter of this chapter. The ideological base of user involvement will be explored as a background to a discussion of the components within the patient–professional relationship which are the ingredients of user involvement. Individual and collective approaches to hearing and releasing the user voice in palliative care are explored. Finally some dilemmas and practice issues in ensuring a strong consumer voice and patient-centred care will be summarized.

## What is it?

The term 'user' has been commonly used in palliative care in relatively recent times. The term is in common parlance in government reports and indicates a degree of choice that recipients of services can exercise in a business model of health care. The term contrasts with the traditional term 'patient' which smacks of a dependent relationship. It relates to 'client' or 'consumer' which also indicate an element of choice. It is important to remember that for many patients they have very little or no opportunity for choice. Also, in a speciality where the holistic, 'total' person approach is key, it is important to remind ourselves that we are talking about *people*: people with unique identities, a range of preferences and characteristics. Although in quality palliative care, however much we would encourage users to be part of an interactive process of assessment and intervention with the professionals in the multi-professional team, many remain, in reality, the compliant object of services (Iskander 1997).

Not all users wish to be involved. However, gradually, we are seeing that as 'users', many patients are divesting themselves of the 'patient' role, are directly seeking personal help, are contributing to the greater well-being, are called to bear witness and are entering the world of giver/provider of care, not just at the receiving end. Additionally, the world of giver/provider of palliative care is inhabited by professionals who frequently will have carer, if not user, experiences themselves, and the value of this component is often underestimated (F. Sheldon, personal communication 2003). Certainly it seems more acceptable for professionals to share their user/carer experience in public forums and teaching.

Far from just being allowed to be the ill and the passive receiver of care and attention, an enlightened and questioning patient population opens up complexity and emphasizes the need for multiprofessional teams carefully to choreograph the delivery of care in conjunction with the patient/carer. The patient's role in the team is changing rapidly, with constant technological developments that have given rise to greater medical and care awareness, possibilities and options. The information revolution through the Internet, and greater public and patient education have accelerated the trend for patients to be *partners* in care where questions are explored, expectations and possibilities discussed (NHS 2006). National organizations and local support and advocacy groups representing different illnesses offer a wide range of information and, in some cases, training for users. Increasingly, the health care professionals surrounding the patient have adopted an empower-ment and advocacy model away from traditional paternalistic approaches (Speck 1998).

In moving away from paternalism in medical care, there is a clear emphasis towards patient autonomy, empowerment and choice, although practice experience would indicate a wide variety of philosophies operating. Some professionals, particularly doctors, are so intent on providing options for treatment or non-treatment that they withhold their own experience or sug-gestions to assist the patient or carer in making a decision, e.g. whether to have surgical intervention for a malignancy or not. This can leave the patient feeling abandoned over decision making (Speck 1998). Speck claims that giving patients the maximum amount of information but withholding your own experience and advice is a very powerful thing to do and can actually disempower them. He remarks that power is not a finite commodity that is in the possession of one party or the other, but it needs sharing to create an acceptable balance for the individual patient/carer. Some patients may indeed want doctors to be paternalistic (Obholtzer 1999).

Coming from a gender perspective on the paternalism–empowerment debate, Davies posits that professionalism is based on traditional male values of detachment, rationality, control, mastery and hierarchical relations that achieve and maintain expert knowledge (Davies 1995). The professional is expected to have the knowledge and to know the answers. It is a shift to not know, to acknowledge this, to ask and to develop a willingness to learn from the patients. For user involvement, we need to develop a different power base. The *relationship* between professional and user becomes the powerbase, rather than our professional expertise. In practice, multiprofessional teams can be very ambivalent about this, particularly in palliative care when one is dealing with a very uncertain world, 'holding' user/carer/one's own anxiety, and the reality is that there is pressure to 'be the expert' in dying.

In the UK, over the last few years, repeated government documents and publications have upheld the patient–professional partnership model and a patient-centred service.

The NHS Plan states, 'patients and citizens will have a greater say in the National Health Service and the provision of services will be centred on patients' needs' (Department of Health 2000). The need for user involvement in the planning, prioritization and delivery of care is explicit in the NHS Cancer Plan (Department of Health 2000). The Department further emphasizes, 'A patient-centred service demands more power for patients. Patient power will be backed by the new operational arrangements we are making to put the patient at the heart of the NHS. Patients will be in the driving seat' (National Council 2004). The challenge for multiprofessional teams is to translate these ideological statements into sound practice that makes a difference to users'/carers' lives.

User involvement is concerned with the meaningful and active participation and consultation of service users in the planning, delivery, development and evaluation of the service at a level they feel comfortable with and from their unique perspective. The level of the involvement must be self-determined by the user concerned and they cannot be expected to represent the community of users, but must be free to represent themselves (see Table 4.1).

Payne *et al.* in a new research report are clear that there is no consensus as to what user involvement is. Payne's research group on user involvement takes it to mean 'the way people, who use public services, are involved in making suggestions and taking decisions about how different services are run and developed. User involvement is about how service users are involved in shaping or building the future of public services' (Payne *et al.* 2005).

The National Institute for Clinical Excellence (NICE) Guidance for adults with cancer, which places user involvement high on the agenda, defines it as:

enabling people who use—or may use—services to voice their experiences and influence broader care. They may participate in:

- service planning to ensure that services meet the needs of patients and carers
- the evaluation of services
- mutual support with other patients and carers through self-help and support groups and individual peer to peer support schemes (NICE 2004, 2.3.).

User involvement is a process of several elements and is not something that happens in a single event. Several strands make up a whole, an entire system of involving users/carers. Tritter *et al.*'s diagrammatic representation of user involvement emphasizes the circular process (see Fig. 4.1).

**Table 4.1** Key elements of good practice in user involvement

Meaningful—beyond tokenism—and that involvement is taken seriously
A power base—practical and emotional support may be needed in empowering users to participate actively
From their own perspective—most users can only talk for themselves; they cannot represent all users
At a level they feel comfortable—their experience may be very different from that of professionals and contributions need to be attuned to their particular experience

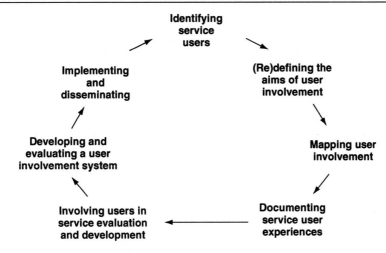

**Fig. 4.1** Cycle of user involvement (Tritter *et al.* 2004).

User involvement can be experienced directly or indirectly at two levels: the individual and/or the collective (Table 4.2). For a true partnership to be established, there needs to be engagement at each level by both team and user.

At a policy level in the UK, the National Health Service (NHS) is quite convinced that the partnership model is desirable. According to Sir Nigel Crisp, former Chief Executive of the NHS, 'the biggest patient benefit, the biggest improvement in health care and the biggest gains from additional funding comes when patients, managers and clinicians work in partnership to redesign clinical processes' (Crisp 2000).

## Pre-requisites to user involvement in the multiprofessional team

### A relationship of trust

To consider the core elements of the relationship between the patient/carers and professionals as team members, there can be no viable interplay and exchange if there is no trust, empathy and genuineness. The patient/carer

**Table 4.2** User involvement: levels of engagement

|            | Direct                       | Indirect                          |
|------------|------------------------------|-----------------------------------|
| Individual | Review of care               | User stories/publication          |
|            | Quality of life questionnaire| Creative arts/expression          |
|            | User–professional discussion | Support group discussion          |
| Collective | User forum/focus group       | Organizational statements         |
|            | Questionnaires/surveys       | Surveys of national organizations |
|            | Individual interviews        | Complaints analyses               |

needs to be heard and understood. They need to be taken seriously and feel safe to explore feelings, thoughts and fears. Regnard quotes Stedeford as stating that a hospice offers 'a safe place to suffer' (C. Regnard, personal communication 1999).

The professional needs to engage the patient/carer in the process of assessment and intervention. The multiprofessional team needs to treat the patient as a person who is capable of understanding the treatment and care on offer, and offer opportunities to receive explanations about drugs, their side effects and how the appropriate doses can be determined in a spirit of collaboration. With an appreciation of the pattern of the intricacies of the administration of morphine, or an application for grants or the trial of a new mattress, for example, the patient/carer is more likely to be engaged in a cooperative venture with the professionals involved.

Some might say that there needs to be some balance and reciprocity in the relationship at all levels. A patient cannot constantly be at the receiving end of the relationship: that by bestowing thanks, gifts or offering to participate in 'user involvement' activities, the patient attempts to give back to the team in some way. As a basis of the trust relationship, the patient and carer need to experience an honest relationship, where the professional is prepared to voice his/her doubts and lack of knowledge to the patient's questions, e.g. is there life after death?'; or 'will I choke to death?' etc. Saunders' words are powerful reminders of this: 'In the last scene between us and death, there is no more pretence' (Saunders 1999).

## A relationship of 'critical friendship'

Can there truly be a balanced relationship of teamwork where users/carers feel comfortable enough to be 'critical friends' of the care or the service, when they are primarily the recipients of care provided by health professionals who may have had hundreds and thousands of patients with similar medical diagnoses and are used to 'diagnosing dying' (Lickiss *et al.* 2004) and watching the process? There is an immediate power imbalance of knowledge and experience. The patient is experiencing their 'journey' for the first and only time with their own set of fears, frustrations and uncertainties. The questions they hold are bound to be qualitatively different from those of the professionals involved. The language used to frame and explain their experiences will be different from that of the professionals involved. The multiprofessional team needs to be attuned to these and other differences that create obstacles in establishing a relationship of critical friendship.

Palliative care, in its support for the fullness of life—body, mind and spirit—and of what makes the individual human, aims to work with the whole person. In naming the nature of the suffering and the resilience that can so often accompany end-of-life care, the multiprofessional team will be eager to identify the nature of the experience for the patient and carers referred. The process of palliative care endeavours to promote discovery, identify the healthy sides of people, facilitate transformation and enhance resilience and coping. A multiprofessional team cannot tap into the inner strengths and personal resources of people without a close partnership.

This partnership can only be reciprocal if permission is given to the patient and carer to be critical, to refuse, to express disappointment and not to be stuck in the 'grateful patient syndrome' (Oliviere *et al.* 1998). Deliberations between professionals and patients must allow for a variety of views: one patient to voice either 'I love day care; it keeps you from thinking you're ill' or 'I don't want to consider day care—all those people talking about their illnesses'. A skilled professional will respect the views expressed, even if misguided, and allow room for change of perspectives and decisions. The relationship must also allow for criticisms when the team does not 'get it right'.

## A 'systemic' relationship

Patient and carer needs are not an entity but a process (Payne 2001). The interdependent, interacting and interconnected nature of patient, carer and professional means that changes in one area will have a knock-on effect on another. For example, a difference of opinion between two health professionals involved—GP and palliative care nurse—being unresolved will tarnish the seamlessness of the service delivered. Multiprofessional teams are dynamic with changing membership, change of status and practices, and cohesion and vigour. The introduction of new audits, clinical outcome scales or research projects will affect users and carers in some way.

Frank, a patient, stresses the interactive nature of professional and carers working together: 'I cannot accept it when medical staff, family and friends fail to recognise that they are participants in the process of illness. Their actions shape the behaviour of the ill person.....' (Frank, 1991).

The relationship between user and professional is a two-way relationship of sustenance. Professionals frequently witness to a strong sense of privilege in being involved in end-of-life care work. When the public and lay view so often is that the work is depressing and distressing, professionals are so often aware of how much they receive in learning, for their own quality of life experiences and the sense of entering a precious world.

We frequently see how both patient and family may find peace and strength for themselves when we know we have given so little. There are possibilities in people facing death that are a constant astonishment. We will see them more often if we can gain the confidence to approach our fellows without hiding behind a professional mask, and meet as one person with another, both aware of the depths of a pain that somehow has its healing within itself. In this discovery we may find out as much about living as about dying. People at the end of their lives will then be our teachers (Saunders 1995).

Organizations, of which individual multiprofessional teams are a part, need to be vigilant of the demands of non-direct patient care time, with increased statutory training and updates or new procedures to be assimilated. This would be reminiscent of the findings in the 1950s of Menzies on how nurses contain anxiety when caring in difficult and distasteful situations. Nurses developed a range of defence mechanisms including depersonalizing patients and the avoidance of decision making and conflict (Menzies 1959). It is also said that staff cannot engage in user involvement if they do not experience involvement and consultation for themselves within their organization. It would seem that a listening organization would be conducive to a staff team with commitment to listening and involving users, but rigorous research needs to be undertaken in this area to ascertain whether this is true.

### A relationship of contradiction, paradox and ambiguity

The patients/carers are centrally located in the basic and fast-changing processes in palliative care. Patients change their viewpoints, preferences and positions in the light of changing symptoms and experiences in the illness journey. We may all be familiar with the despondent patient who takes the viewpoint of 'you wouldn't let a dog suffer' but who is full of plans when symptoms are well controlled.

The dimensions of contradiction and paradox are common: acknowledging–denying; hoping yet despairing; talking–remaining silent; receiving help yet rejecting it; desiring intimacy–distance; making future plans–staying in the past/present; collapsing and disconnected or remaining connected and resilient; these are all phenomena the professionals are working with, as will the patient/carers. Saunders reminds us, 'the window to suffering can be a window to peace and opportunity' (Saunders 2001). These common paradoxes in palliative care can only be worked in partnership, where empathy is given and received. Feedback, including helplessness, is two way, and ways forward need to be honestly explored (Speck 1994).

As professionals in teams, one needs to be reflective, aware of the evidence base of practice yet engage with the agendas of service users and carers, making space to invite their views. This draws on a set of skills of negotiation with service users at an individual care level, and discussions around uncertainty may conflict with expectations 'to know how it is going to be and what's best.'

### A consumer relationship

Repeatedly cancer patients claim that they wish to be treated as people and not patients. In the 1980s, as the AIDS epidemic loomed in North America and Europe, articulate patients heightened the consumer voice in treatment and care. Examples of user participation multiplied as with development of the

London Lighthouse (Oliviere *et al.* 1998) and other HIV/AIDS facilities. Beresford *et al.* comment on the emerging 'management/consumerist approach' to user involvement from the 1980s (Beresford *et al.* 2005). The business ethic has permeated health care and, in some models of care, 'the customer is always right'; much time is spent assessing user satisfaction and handling complaints to ensure standards of service are maintained high. With a degree of competitiveness for funding—be it government or community fundraising—palliative care teams and organizations are inevitably in a degree of service competitiveness, with a pride and keenness to display their 'wares', e.g. out of hours service, sitters at home, top of the range beds, etc. Although consumers do not always have a choice as to which service they will use or not, services are in a consumerist relationship with other teams and organizations.

Certainly the consumer movement has played an important role in how professionals and teams understand bereavement (Silverman 2005). The number of self-help groups and organizations has grown, user groups facilitated by national organizations (e.g. Help the Hospices, Macmillan and Cruse Bereavement Care) multiplied and there is a volume of consumers and bereaved people who have set up services or developed theoretical perspectives following their experiences, e.g. bereaved parents.

Silverman reminds us that 'grief is a universal human experience; everyone needs to be an expert' (Silverman 2005).

### *A relationship of patient–professional partnership*

Palliative care has encouraged a 'levelling' of patient and professional, based on needs and wishes; verbal and non-verbal communications; and integrating as much as possible carers' needs and preferences. The professional does not have a magical set of skills to be used on unthinking patients and carers. Rather, the professional brings rich knowledge and skills and essentially experience that is negotiated with the ill person's unique experience, needs and wishes. These are blended together to work out a consistency of response that is required in the specific case. In a sense, a joint reflection process has to be promoted within the culture of the patient–professional relationship: a joint empathic exploration of the issues in the hope that the final decision reached will be one where all parties can feel committed. Good and attentive listening is not user involvement but the means by which the multiprofessional team may achieve it.

Partnership has evolved from one of 'doctor knows best' through 'multi-professional team knows best' to 'patient–professional partnership is best'. It is now not uncommon for a patient and GP to sit together looking at findings on the Internet on a patient's condition and to discuss it, examining possibilities in partnership. Jenkins notes that, 'increasingly it is seen as desirable for persons with a terminal illness and their carers not only to understand more about the nature, cause and mechanisms of a disease, but also to take an active part in making decisions about treatment' (Jenkins 2000).

### A 'required' relationship

In the UK, with the change of culture in requiring user involvement in health care, the multiprofessional team has had to adapt to a new emphasis on recording attempts to survey and record user views, as part of quality assurance and clinical governance. This has taken the form of questionnaires, audits, complaints analysis, user forums and focus groups.

More recently, the NICE Guidance on Supportive and Palliative Care has recommended that 'mechanisms should be established to enable the views of people with cancer and their carers to influence the development, delivery and evaluation of cancer services' (NICE 2004). User involvement, as one of the main themes of the NICE Guidance, further states that, 'patients want to be treated as individuals, with dignity and respect, and to have their voices heard in decisions about treatment and care. Should they need it, they expect to be offered optimal symptom control and psychological, social and spiritual support. They want to be assured that their families and carers will receive support during their illness' (NICE 2004). This makes it very clear to service providers that both at an individual patient care and at a collective level, user involvement is crucial.

Accompanying the government emphasis on user involvement is a whole new structure to increase patient and public involvement, including patient advocacy and liaison services, patient forums, an independent complaints advocacy service and liaison arrangements between the health and social services sectors. There is a whole new sector within the NHS to facilitate public and patient participation in services. Multiprofessional teams need to be familiar with local arrangements.

## How to capture the voice of the user when expressed individually or collectively

### Individual and advocacy role

'You matter because you are you and you matter to the last moment of your life. We will do all we can to help you, not only to die peacefully but to live until you die' (Saunders 1976). Recognizing people are whole human beings, even if very ill, also implies they have rights and responsibilities, and expectations between user and professional do not get automatically waived because the patient is dying.

Thirty years after Saunders wrote the above, we have a major national palliative care agenda to improve access for all individual, groups and communities (Oliviere and Monroe 2004). Furthermore, it is recognized that the patient is an 'expert' and the most knowledgeable on his/her body and condition. In the sphere of chronic illness, for example, the government has launched the 'Expert Patients' Programme which is a self-management course giving people the confidence, skills and knowledge to manage long-term health conditions better (Expert Patients 2006).

To consider aspects of the individual voice and what some of the complexities are, let us reflect on the scenario given in Box 4.1. In this patient and carer story, there remain many elements which would need to be taken into account for the patient and carer to be effective members of the team, not just in name.

Palliative care teams and professionals can make mistakes; the important outcome is that there is recognition, review and learning from the incident.

● The need to listen, hear and recognize the feedback which belongs to the user/carer, whilst not becoming defensive by labelling through interpretation, e.g. 'you are angry'. It may be true that the reaction is part of a patient/carer's unrecognized anger, but this interpretation needs recognizing as

---

**Box 4.1** ERICA AND RICK

Erica, in her sixties, with advanced ovarian cancer entered a hospice for end of life care. Loss, change and bereavement were not foreign to her. What of Erica's background in understanding her care in the hospice and of the past working in the present? Erica, was completely blind and so was her husband, Rick. They had no children.

Erica arrived in the UK, a 12-year-old Jewish girl from Austria at the outbreak of the Second World War, sent by her parents, not on the Kinderstransport but organised by the Jewish Blind Society. Her parents planned to follow but never arrived. Erica arrived with a placard around her neck giving her name and language she spoke. Not a word of English.

She was brought up in a residential school for the blind, was a very bright student and wanted to go to university and train as a social worker. However, she was discouraged from doing this but nevertheless studied modern languages at the London School of Economics, including a year at the Sorbonne in Paris. Just prior to admission to the hospice, Erica was head of modern languages in a secondary school.

Transferred from hospital to the hospice, Erica had laid out all her things over her bed to manage her environment but the next day a member of staff entered her room and told Erica 'we mustn't have things on the bed; when visitors come in, it looks bad'. The staff member tidied up Erica's possessions onto her bedside locker, without explaining to her where each thing was.

Erica was upset and remained 'thrown' by this incident for the 3 week stay at the hospice before she died. She did not feel cared for or in control. Rick was grateful for the medical treatment, but not impressed by the care given and Erica died unhappy.

Rick continued to be very troubled by his wife's distress. In his words, 'she had felt ignored and excluded'. Some weeks later, he went to see the Nursing Director and was told (or at least that was his understanding) that Erica was an angry person and that it was very natural for him, too, to be angry in bereavement. To date, Rick ruminates on this incident and it remains a distinct feature in his bereavement.

Firth *et al.* (2005)—reproduced with permission.

---

belonging to the professionals and must not be taken away from the patient/carer experience.
- There are implications for 'making it safe' for the user/carer to comment without resorting to formal mechanisms to express complaint.
- The opportunities to use user feedback mechanisms and experience to improve services.

Toynbee's user-centred statement on bereavement applies to all aspects of patient/carer care: 'there is only one obvious lesson to learn from other people's grief—to believe what they say about it' (Toynbee, 1996).

### The collective voice

Patients and carers contribute to the multiprofessional team through the collectivity of their writings, through the creative arts, speaking and teaching, to specific participation on working groups of advisory or executive nature and in evaluation and feedback. There are numerous ways in which patients and carers have contributed their experiences and unique perspectives to the multiprofessional team. It is now common to invite users to comment on drafts of leaflets and literature to be published with the user perspective. Tritter *et al.* (2004) give one of the best explorations of the methods and ways of documenting cancer service users' experiences.

Arnstein's 'ladder of participation' stresses the different levels of involvement from consultation, where professionals are in control, to full participation, where users have more control of the agenda and options available and a user–professional partnership is at work (Arnstein 1969).

In a recent research report, Payne *et al.* (2005) summarize the many levels of involvement from tokenism and potential manipulation to empowerment and user-led services. Hoyes *et al.* (1993) have proposed a dimension from high to low involvement.

HIGH
- Users have authority to make decisions
- Users have authority to make selected decisions
- Users' views are sought before decisions are finalized
- Users may take the initiative to influence decisions
- Decisions are publicized and explained before implementation
- Information is given about decisions made.

LOW

It is certainly important to be clear for what purpose the involvement is to be and to gear methods accordingly. For example, to ascertain users' views on food provision, a focus group and combination of questionnaire and individual interview feedback may be quite sufficient. However, for ideas on how users can more meaningfully be involved within an organization or team, a series of forum meetings with facilitation and an open discussion with a range of service users and staff may be more appropriate. In the latter, the power base of the service users needs to be firm enough to produce meaningful dialogue.

## Service users in education and reflective practice for staff

For a long time now, patients and more recently carers have been recording their experiences (Clark *et al.* 2005) through many forms of writing: their stories and narratives, creative writing, letters and articles. The insights these can give a multiprofessional team, combined with the messages from what seems an increasing range of media available to individuals patients, can give powerful messages. In day care settings, there appear to be a range of opportunities for users to record thoughts and feelings, including painting, use of clay, drama and video-making. Although the primary purpose is therapeutic or to leave memories for loved ones, nevertheless the data captured can help further understandings of facets of the patient experience. Indeed some of these creative experiences are often interpreted as 'user involvement'.

Referring to working with patients with amyotrophic lateral sclerosis (motor neuron disease), Saunders writes, 'all the knowledge acquired since the early days ....serves above all to help people to belong, however profound their losses, and to continue to teach us the endurance we can only admire and from which we continue to learn' (Saunders, 2000). Indeed, Saunders has always modelled an approach that placed the patient not only at the centre of decision-making processes (Kirkham 1998) but also in teaching.

Service users have for a long time written accounts of their experiences (Clark 2005) and continue to do so as well as chair, speak at conferences and ask pertinent questions at meetings. Numerous websites give personal accounts and helpful information from individuals, patient groups or national organizations. One among many is the DIPEx website, sharing personal experiences of health and illness, including living with dying and palliative care (DIPEx.org 2005).

One interesting education project is the 'goldfish bowl' method of teaching fifth year medical students about patient experiences and the illness journey. The session involves the group of day centre patients and a facilitator sitting in an inner circle, the medical students forming an outer circle. The facilitator engages the patients in a 20 min discourse on the range of hospice services, and the impact of these services on the patients, their carers' quality of life and functioning (Edmonds 2004). The students can then intervene and ask the patients' questions. The patients feel this is a safe and non-threatening teaching environment. The goldfish bowl session is consistently extremely well evaluated.

*Service users and evaluation*

Higginson, referring to the World Health Organization's definition of evaluation, describes it as, 'the systematic and scientific study of determining whether a therapy or service is successful in achieving pre-determined goals' (Higginson 1999).

The particular evaluation for the palliative care patient and carer is that they may not have had pre-determined goals but have lived and adapted to the experience of illness. This is the unique element in feedback that they can bring to the evaluation process: the lived experience and the qualitative feedback to accompany quantitative measures. For example, the amount of breakthrough pain may be less, as reported in one evaluative project, the challenge of managing the medications reported by the patients being more complex.

Quinn, commenting on involving users in research, states that 'users perspectives on evaluation challenge the reliance on standardized outcomes' (Quinn 2005). She quotes Fisher who emphasized the importance of process, the nature of relationships between staff and service users: 'no good outcomes without good process' (Fisher 2002).

Users are increasingly being actively involved in research beyond the role of subjects; in writing proposals, evaluating them, on steering and advisory groups and in using the findings (Hanley 2005). The North Trent Cancer Research Network Consumer Research Panel, whose Chair and Vice-chairs are a service user and carer, was formed under the auspices of the Academic Unit of Supportive Care at the University of Sheffield and is an outstanding example of users, carers and researchers working together. The panel is involved with all stages of research and there are regular conferences on service users and researchers (North Trent Cancer Research Panel 2005).

*Service users as auditors and inspectors*

As has been recognized, patients relate to a number of different teams, including primary care teams of GPs, community nurses, health visitors and a range of health professionals to whom the team have access, e.g. counsellors, psychologists, dietician, physiotherapist, etc.

A good example is the Improving Practice Questionnaire (IPQ), a patient-focused approach to measure primary care practitioner and practice performance, from the point of view of patients (Greco and Carter 2002). The patient spends a considerable amount of time as part of the primary care team. Dixon claims that the IPQ will become part of GP appraisal and revalidation, which underlines the emphasis and influence on user feedback (Dixon 2002). The challenging assessment tool has led to some practices sharing the results with patient focus or 'critical friend' groups. In some practices, Dixon claims some far-reaching developments have been initiated: 'this is leading to a new relationship between the practice and its patients, which goes far beyond simply pointing out where the practice is going wrong or right. It has led to real involvement of patients in the services that the practice offers. This could be the beginning of a new partnership between patients and health professionals, which will enable the whole local community to look after itself better' (Dixon 2002).

The other example is from specialist palliative care at St Christopher's Hospice, London. Some years ago, the Education and Training Department initiated a 'Users' Education Advisory Group', a group of nine users and bereaved carers, chaired by a carer, who meet with the Director of Education and Training quarterly. The aim of the group is to attend, sample, monitor and report on the education courses to ensure that the courses are patient-centred and that 'the patient is always present in the classroom' (Lishman and Oliviere 2004; Firth *et al.* 2005). It clearly attracts users who have a background or interest in education, from a professor in psychiatry, a health visitor and a GP, but also users who have never directly been involved in education before. Members of the group occasionally present and chair study days in St Christopher's Education Centre and suggest topics for the education programme. For example, issues for men were suggested, members of the group helping in identifying suitable speakers. The group forms part of the education and training quality assurance activities complementing student evaluations and teacher peer observations. The group has been involved in a slight shift in practice in the Education Centre where it is now commonplace to find users/carers registered for courses on delegates' lists. What is more challenging is delegates finding they are sitting next to a user.

## Managing collective user involvement

Although published research in user involvement in palliative care is extremely limited on models and effective outcomes, practice from various experiences of user involvement indicates certain basic 'lessons learned' (Kraus *et al* 2003).

### Process is important

How the services users are welcomed and put at ease; opportunities to 'tell their story'; nursing and other support; feeling valued to the extent of feeding back decisions and changes which have resulted from the involvement, all these are integral to the successful outcome of any user involvement event.

### Boundaries

Safe boundaries in maintaining confidentiality between clinical discussions and examples of care (or lack of) given in a user consultation event need maintaining.

In one hospice, non-clinical staff conduct the User Forum to ensure separation between clinical discussions and service improvement consultations.

### Briefing and training of staff—and users

It is essential that staff understand the nature of user involvement and support its aims, otherwise inadvertent undermining can occur. In addition, the success of user involvement is dependent in part on the enthusiasm of staff in inviting users and explaining the nature of the commitment. If staff and team members are not convinced of the value—or only see the work as a 'tick box' exercise to go through the motions of 'doing' user involvement—then the impact will be diluted.

Preparation and explanation for users and carers on key terms and jargon; the structure of the organization or team; how change and decision making occur; how to make their voice heard; and financial and practical considerations in being involved are amongst areas to clarify with those being included in user involvement activities.

### Opportunities to 'leave a legacy'

One strong motivating factor for patients and carers in participating in user involvement seems to be the fulfilment in feeling their experience is helping others in the future and that even negative experiences are harnessed positively to improve services. Research needs to be undertaken in what motivates and in understanding the satisfactions for users in being involved.

## The benefits of user involvement

The benefits and limitations of user involvement will be very different if we are considering involvement at individual clinical care level or service improvement level (see Table 4.3).

## The challenges of user involvement

There are a number of challenges and obstacles to overcome to facilitate effective user involvement. Table 4.4 summarizes these.

Some users and carers need advocacy to empower them when considering individualized best care. For example, interpreters who are suitably trained and supported are needed for those whose first language is not English. Further, research suggests that only 54 per cent of people with learning disabilities attend their parents' funerals (Blackman 2003). Knowing this, professionals

**Table 4.3** The benefits of user involvement

For the user
    More likely to meet their individual needs
    Feel valued
    Empowered
    Respected
    Autonomous
    Best use of team resources
    Develops better coping strategies
    Satisfaction of 'leaving a legacy'
    Illness has greater meaning
For the professional
    Satisfaction of 'getting it right'
    Time efficient
    Better informed user group
    More likely to get informed consent
    Better shared decision making
    Users' wishes more integrated with care plan
    More compassionate response to need
For the organization
    Services used better
    Improved clinical governance
    Good risk management
    Services better planned to respond to need
    Reassurance that you are 'getting it right'
    Better balanced partnership

Based on Iskander (1997).

need to be extra vigilant to ensure carers with learning disabilities have an opportunity to participate in funerals, with all the preparation, family negotiation and anxiety holding that this may involve.

As trends towards greater user involvement in service improvement and evaluation become more pronounced, users have been known to carry out a useful function of expressing the views of professionals, e.g. in emphasizing

**Table 4.4** Challenges and obstacles to user involvement

Staff feel criticized and become defensive; conflict over dual roles of clinical responsibilities and service development
User fears that treatment will be adversely affected
Users do not have wider clinical experience or the organizational 'bigger picture' regarding resources
Easy to 'go through the motions' of involvement without effective change
Users' main preoccupation is their individual situation, not beyond
Costly in time, money and skill
Needs management commitment and a culture of user involvement
Reaching a variety of users
Conflicting perspectives amongst service users
Service users who do not wish to be involved
Training for staff and users—user involvement involves changes in perspectives and practices
Access to 'unheard minorities'
Users' dependence on and dominance of carers' voices
Users' and professional doubts of 'will it change anything?'

the need for more day centre places, website improvements or the need for providing diversity in catering. As user involvement has become high profile for organizations, a request expressed by the user group may be seen as acceptable and to outweigh staff demands. This can be seen as another way of users and professionals working together, which may be used positively or negatively. For example, a small group of day centre members in one hospice were due to be 'discharged' to make room for newly referred patients. This had caused much concern on the part of clinical staff and the patients due for discharge and resulted in vociferous complaints to senior management from a small group of users. The result was the provision of facilities with a small amount of staff input to initiate a self-help facility for day centre patients who were relatively well.

## Ethical considerations

The team will experience the many ongoing ethical dilemmas involved in sensitive individual patient care: to tell or not to tell; to treat or not to treat; conflict between carer and patient re discharge or over accepting additional help; and issues of communication, confidentiality, competence and consent (see Chapter 11 of this volume). At the core of user involvement is the debate over the appropriateness of paternalism, which has ethical implications. 'To be paternalistic involves both forming a judgment about what's best for another individual and then seeking to impose that judgment' (Boyd *et al.* 1997). How a professional negotiates with a patient what's best and what's preferential, given the professional training and experience of the professional, can lead to real dilemmas.

All of these can be influenced by culture and ethnicity. For example, in general terms, North American and north-west European culture emphasizes patient autonomy, and this influences practice in imparting information on diagnosis. However, in southern Europe, the tendency is for families to filter what information is given to the patient (Nunez Olarte 2003). In other cultures and religions, male members of the community might monitor and control what the female patient might receive in the way of care and treatment. These can pose real concerns and dilemmas for multiprofessional teams in establishing an integration of acceptable professional practice, professional values and patient/carer choice. In the AIDS field in the UK, it is noted that some patients from Africa prefer a paternalist medical approach (see Box 4.2).

The common ethical concerns related to collective user involvement include issues of respect for the user/carer and providing necessary support if they feel upset by the process of user involvement, informed consent and handling data (Tritter *et al.* 2004). What follows are some specific ethical

---

**Box 4.2** MRS M

---

Mrs M was a patient with cancer of the breast and extensive secondaries. She was married and had two adult unemployed children in their twenties at home. The family were from India. The home care palliative care team became very divided as Mrs M's condition was deteriorating and the family did not recognize that she was no longer able to cope with the cleaning, shopping and cooking. In view of Mrs M's continuing efforts to complete all the household tasks without input from the family, it was assessed that home help should be introduced to maintain her functioning. The husband and son were seen to be blocking attempts made by the nurse to introduce home help but were unwilling to provide the additional help themselves.

---

concerns identified from emerging user involvement developments in palliative care, which have implications for team working.

### The 'professional' patient

This is involvement of a user repeatedly, for consultation or for teaching, who may be distanced from their patient experience as they are in remission and well enough to attend meetings. These users often meet the requirements of agencies to include a service user, but it is not infrequently found that they are no longer in reception of active palliative care. For their part, they often build a career on user involvement activities, finding new satisfactions and outlets for their new energies. This is not to diminish their motives, but they do throw up the need for organizations to consider the most appropriate users to be involved. Issues of self-determination and who defines whether the person is appropriate as a 'user' or not come into play here.

### Exploitation of service users

This relates to the overuse of the same service users for panels, consultation and education for the reasons as stated above and for organizational convenience. Some teams are careful to involve only the same users on a limited number of occasions.

It is important to recognize that inviting service users to participate in education can potentially lead to negative critical comment from audience feedback, although it is the author's experience that users' teaching is generally well evaluated. Preparation and support are essential.

### Critical feedback rebounding on care

Service users can be vulnerable to the extent of feeling pressured to give complimentary feedback and avoid critical comment, lest it affect their current or future care and treatment. It is important to emphasize the anonymity of reporting back and the collective nature of feedback/comment in terms of capturing themes.

## Boundaries

There are several boundary issues that can interfere in user involvement. There have been incidents where veiled criticism of a health professional is prematurely fed back from a user meeting. Before proper discussion has ensued, the individual professional becomes defensive and reluctant to take on board the feedback. Those receiving feedback need to be careful as to how it is relayed.

Issues of confidentiality are sometimes specific to some user involvements, e.g. where a service user is a Trustee. Often those working with user groups may be tempted to share explanations and a rationale for developments or future plans which not all members of an organization are yet party to, e.g. staff changes or financial concerns.

Boundaries around service users expressing discriminatory remarks, e.g. sexist or racist, which would not be tolerated by colleagues need to be tackled sensitively.

One user in a meeting on the change of use of palliative care team resources declared that 'the medical director is a waste of space'. Do the same expectations of behaviour for meetings operate for users as they do for professionals?

## Self-determination

This relates to professionals respecting the self-determination by users, e.g. to conduct meetings on a Saturday when professionals mainly do not work, or requesting change where the team is not convinced of its value. In a particular hospice, the User Forum requested that prayer requests be made public by putting them on the wall to be more visible. Negotiation with the chaplaincy team and good explanation as to why this was inappropriate resolved the issue.

## User representativeness

There is often concern that a user on a committee or group is not representative of the body of users. Can effective user involvement operate if the user or users concerned cannot consult or speak for wider interests? A user can essentially only speak for him/herself and from their unique experience.

It is important to attract enough service users to a project so that a range of interests and perspectives can be voiced. Increasing concerns have been expressed for improved access to palliative care from the most disadvantaged groups (Oliviere and Monroe 2004).

*Payment*

User involvement is not a cheap option, and involves staff time and support costs for user involvement events such as travel and the cost of sitters if carers are attending. Some users have raised payment in lieu of the time they spend on consultation activities, recognizing the imbalance with professionals paid to engage with user involvement activities. Issues of exploitation and possible double standards need to be considered.

## Conclusions

The development of the user involvement movement has heightened the complexity of the planning, provision and evaluation of palliative care services, whether at an individual or a collective level. Every multiprofessional needs to take account of the nature of user involvement, its dimensions and its potential. User involvement involves engaging with the whole experience of patients/carers and understanding their perspectives on their own individual care and/or the service. It can tap into the healthy sides of people and balance the tendency for one-way traffic in the patient–professional partnership (Monroe and Oliviere 2003).

There are specific challenges for team involvement with palliative care users and carers in view of the rapidly changing nature of the illness, the short-term intensity of the contact and the once-only nature of the life event.

Finally, the pressure on palliative care professionals to 'get it right' as it is a 'once only' for the patient and carers can increase stress but also provides rewards in tailoring services and care to meet individual need. Awareness that 'the dissatisfied dead cannot noise abroad the negligence they have experienced' (Hinton, 1972) can also motivate professionals to promote effective and useful user involvement in the service provided by the palliative care team.

## References

Arnstein S (1969). A ladder of citizen participation. *Journal of the American Institute of Planners* **35**, 216–224.

Beresford P, Croft S, Adshead L, Walker J and Wilman K (2005). Involving service users in palliative care: from theory to practice. In: Firth P, Luff G and Oliviere D, ed. *Loss, Change and Bereavement in Palliative Care*. Open University Press, Maidenhead, UK.

Blackman N (2003). *Loss and Learning Disability*. Worth Publishing Ltd, London.

Boyd KM, Higgs R and Pinching AJ (1997). *The New Dictionary of Medical Ethics*. BMJ Publishing Group, London.

Clark D, Thomas C, McDermott E, Bingley A, Payne S and Seymour J (2005). What are the views of people affected by cancer and other illnesses about end of life issues?

*Professional and Patient Perspectives.* International Observatory on End of Life Care, Institute of Health Research, Lancaster University, Lancaster, UK.

Crisp N (2002). *Managing for Excellence in the NHS.* (October). Department of Health, London.

Davies C (1995). *Gender and the Professional Predicament in Nursing.* Open University Press, Milton Keynes, UK.

Department of Health (2000). *The National Cancer Plan.* Department of Health, London.

DIPEx (2005). Personal experiences of health and illness. www.dipex.org. Consulted 24 May 2005.

Dixon M (2002). Foreword. In: Greco M and Carter M. *Improving Practice Questionnaire (IPQ) Tool Kit. A Tool Kit for General Practice.* Aeneas Press, Chichester, UK.

Edmonds P, Burman R and Sinnott C (2004). The goldfish bowl. *European Journal of Palliative Care* 11(2), 69–71.

Expert Patients' Programme (2006). wwwexpertpatients.nhs.uk. Consulted 16 February 2006.

Firth P, Luff G and Oliviere D (2005). *Loss, Change and Bereavement in Palliative Care.* Open University Press, Maidenhead, UK.

Fisher M (2002). The role of service users in problem formulation and technical aspects of social research. *Social Work Education* 21, 305–312.

Frank A (1991). *At the Will of the Body: Reflections of Illness.* Houghton Mifflin, Boston, MA.

Greco M and Carter M (2002). *Improving Practice Questionnaire (IPQ) Tool Kit. A Tool Kit for General Practice.* Aeneas Press, Chichester, UK.

Hanley B (2005). *Research as Empowerment?* Report of a series of seminars organised by the Toronto Group. Joseph Rowntree Foundation, York, UK.

Higginson IR (1999). Paper in National Seminar 'Palliative care. Developing user involvement, improving quality'. In: Beresford P, Broughton F, Croft S, Fouquet S, Oliviere D and Rhodes P, ed. *Palliative Care: Developing User Involvement, Improving Quality.* Brunel University, Middlesex, UK.

Hinton J (1972). *Dying,* 2nd edn. Penguin, Harmondsworth, UK.

Hoyes L, Jeffers S, Lart R, Means R and Taylor M (1993). *User Empowerment and the Reform of Community Care.* School for Advanced Urban Studies, Bristol, p. 9

Iskander R (1997). User involvement: from principles to practice. *Health Visitor* 70, 455–457.

Jenkins P (2000). The internet and the expectations of palliative care consumers. *Progress in Palliative Care* 8, 269–270.

Lamerton R (1986). *East End Doc.* Lutterworth, Cambridge.

Kraus F, Levy J and Oliviere D (2003). Brief report on user involvement at St Christopher's Hospice. *Palliative Medicine* 17, 375–377.

Kirkham S (1998). Editor's note. *Palliative Medicine* 12, 146.

Lickiss JN, Turner KS and Pollock ML (2004). The interdisciplinary team. In: Doyle D, Hanks GFK, Cherny N and Calman K, ed. *Oxford Textbook of Palliative Medicine,* 3rd edn. Oxford University Press, Oxford, pp. 42–46.

Lishman A and Oliviere D (2004). *Users' Education Advisory Group. Brief.* St Christopher's Hospice, London.

Menzies I (1959). *The Functioning of Social Systems as a Defence Against Anxiety.* Tavistock Institute of Human Relations, London.

Monroe B and Oliviere D (2003). *Patient Participation in Palliative Care. A Voice for the Voiceless*. Oxford University Press, Oxford.

National Council for Palliative Care (2004). *Listening to Users*. NCPC, London.

NHS-National Health Service UK (2006). Our health, our care, our say: a new direction in community services. [downloadable from: www.expertpatients.nhs.uk]

NICE (2004). *Guidance on Improving Supportive and Palliative Care for Adults with Cancer*. National Institute for Clinical Excellence, London.

North Trent Cancer Research Network Consumer Research Panel (2005). www.ntcrp. org.uk. Consulted 26 May 2005

Nunez-Olarte J (2003). Cultural aspects of palliative care. In: Monroe B and Oliviere D, ed. *Patient Participation in Palliative Care*. Oxford University Press, Oxford.

Obholtzer A (1999). It takes two to patronise/be patronised. Letter. *Britush Medical Journal* 24 September. http://bmj.bmjjournals.com/cgi/eletters/319/7212/719.

Oliviere D (2001). User involvement in palliative care services. *European Journal of Palliative Care* 8, 238–241.

Oliviere D and Monroe B (2004). *Death, Dying and Social Differences*. Oxford University Press, Oxford.

Oliviere D, Hargreaves R and Monroe B (1998). *Good Practices in Palliative Care: A Psychosocial Perspective*. Ashgate, Aldershot, UK.

Payne S (2001). Paper presented at: Bereavement Research Forum, Oxford, 15 November.

Payne S, Gott M, Small N, Oliviere D, Sargeant A and Young EL (2005). *User Involvement in Palliative Care: A Scoping Study*. University of Sheffield and St Christopher's Hospice, UK. pp. 1–17.

Quinn A (2005). The context of loss, change and bereavement in palliative care. In: Firth P, Luff G and Oliviere D, ed. *Loss, Change and Bereavement in Palliative Care*. Open University Press, Maidenhead, UK, pp. 1–17.

Saunders C (1976). Care of the dying—1. The problem of euthanasia. *Nursing Times* 72, 1003–1005.

Saunders C (1995). Foreword. In: Kearney M, *Mortally Wounded: Stories of Soul Pain, Death and Healing*. Marino Press, Dublin.

Saunders C (1999). 'Windows on suffering'. Lecture at the Trent Palliative Care Centre, Sheffield, UK (June).

Saunders C (2000). Foreword. In: Oliver D, Borasio GD and Walsh D, ed. *Palliative Care in Amyotrophic Lateral Sclerosis*. Oxford University Press, Oxford.

Saunders C (2001). Foreword. In: Ferrell BR and Coyle N, ed. *Palliative Nursing*. Oxford University Press, Oxford.

Silverman PR (2005). Mourning: a changing view. In: Firth P, Luff G and Oliviere D, ed. *Loss, Change and Bereavement in Palliative Care*. Open University Press, Maidenhead, UK, pp. 18–37.

Small N (2005). User voices in palliative care. In: Faull C, Carter Y and Daniels L, ed. *Handbook of Palliative Care*, 2nd edn. Blackwell Publishing, Oxford.

Small N and Rhodes P (2000). *Too Ill to Talk? User Involvement and Palliative Care*. Routledge, London.

Speck P (1994). Working with dying people. On being good enough. In: Obholzer A and Roberts V, ed. *The Unconscious at Work. Individuals and Organisational Stress in the Human Services*. Routledge, London.

Speck P (1998). Power and autonomy in palliative care: a matter of balance. Editorial. *Palliative Medicine* **12**, 145–146.

Toynbee P (1996). Patient and carer perspective. Cited in: Oliviere D, Hargreaves R and Monroe B. (1998) *Good Practices in Palliative Care: A Psychosocial Perspective*. Ashgate, Aldershot, UK, p. 11

Tritter J, Daykin N, Evans S, and Sanidas M (2004). *Improving Cancer Services Through Patient Involvement*. Radcliffe Medical Press, Abingdon, UK.

# 5

# Leaders and followers

*Peter Speck*

A great deal has been written about leadership in organizations, but very little attention is paid to the importance of followership. A shepherd without sheep, however troublesome they may be at times, will have a rather lonely and unfulfilled existence. The inter-relatedness of leader and follower is crucial in the life of any team or enterprise if the primary task is to be achieved. Similarly, the way in which leaders and followers relate will influence not only the team dynamic but also the use, or abuse, of power and authority within the work setting. Those who work in an interdisciplinary way will find that there are times when they move out of the leadership role to become a follower, and vice versa. The emotional and psychological health of the team will to a large extent depend on the ease with which these transitions occur as different disciplines take the lead in the planning and provision of care at various points along the patient pathway. In this chapter, I wish to explore some of these issues and their importance for the dynamic that operates within the team, between teams and within the wider organization, and implications for the relationship between professional carer and patient.

## Leadership

In our present age, leadership has come to be associated more with inspiration, vision and the ability to relate to others, than with orders and commands. It is primarily concerned with a relationship through which one person is able to influence the behaviour of others. Leadership is a social process through which one person, for example a team leader, harnesses the knowledge, skills and motivation of other team members in order to achieve an agreed task. In the case of palliative care, this is the delivery of quality care to patients and families. In order to achieve the desired outcome, the leader has to influence the actions of the team in the desired direction, to meet any reasonable individual needs, and manage the requirements of the task itself. Thus leadership is related to motivation, communication and interpersonal behaviour.

## Motivation

Motivation is what makes people act or behave the way they do. It begins with the various needs that exist within us all which we seek to satisfy in either our personal, our social or our work life. If these needs are unsatisfied, we establish a goal—consciously or unconsciously—and take action to achieve that goal. Within the context of work, this is one of the prime reasons for people engaging or devoting more time to tasks that are not necessarily matched to the primary task of the organization. This can be described as an 'as if' task, and potentially leads to off-task activity (see Chapter 7 of this volume).

Motivation is a forward-looking process and, therefore, is more about expectations than about satisfactions. The expectations held by people at work may not always be clearly acknowledged or expressed, and may, at times, be unrealistic in terms of the individual's skill and ability, or the scope provided by the role occupied within the team or organization. People are usually only motivated if they think they will get what they want, or perhaps avoid what they do not want. A key factor in motivation is the expectation of reward, which is not necessarily in terms of money.

The value of rewards to the individual is related to the likelihood of the reward satisfying the individual's need for security, social esteem and self-fulfilment. To be effective, a reward needs to be commensurate with the effort required, as perceived by the individual, to perform the task. The demands of the organization, as expressed through management, may require effort beyond the capacity of the individual, and outside of the individual's ability to control the pace and volume of the workload. This is a frequent cause of work-related stress (see Chapter 7 of this volume).

Other factors affecting motivation include:

- Perceptions about the job—how clearly is the required task understood?
- Ability—does the individual believe she/he has the necessary skills, knowledge?
- Influence of others—group pressures, family (which may be positive or negative), the need to achieve or prove oneself
- The work itself—does it give satisfaction, opportunities for achievement and responsibility?

The concerns of motivation and reward are important factors for leaders to be aware of if they are to be able to 'knit' together a varied range of people, skills and knowledge into a healthy functioning team. Communication within the team is vital to this process and needs to be sufficiently open to sanction discussion of factors relating to motivation, expectation, emotional agenda and the interpersonal dynamics associated with team working. For this to happen, it can be helpful for the leader to:

- understand the needs of staff
- understand what they want
- differentiate between needs and wants
- assess whether the financial rewards are appropriate
- consider recognition, praise, promotion
- review expectations, and whether these are achievable
- review levels of responsibility of team members
- recognize that group pressure can affect motivation for good or ill
- not ignore unconscious processes—they affect the leader too!

Leadership requires considerable ability to be sensitive and discerning of the various needs and wants of team members as well as good communication skills to listen and respond appropriately to both the individual and the team as a whole, while also maintaining a clear focus on the task and vision.

### Leader and/or manager

In the context of palliative care, leadership can often be complicated further by the leader having also to exercise a management function. There can be a tension between these two functions, especially if the person concerned does not make it clear to others what role he/she is taking up at any particular time. In many ways, the management role can be seen as focusing on planning, organizing, directing and controlling the activities of others, whereas leadership gives more attention to communicating with, motivating and encouraging other people through involvement (Levine and Crom 1994). Balancing these two roles in terms of time can be difficult in a busy work setting. Much confusion and hurt can be experienced where the leader, when taking up a management role, has to follow through a disciplinary procedure with a team member who fails to recognize the change in role, task and behaviour in the leader. This has sometimes been the experience of ward managers leading a ward team of nurses, who may enjoy a friendly personal and social relationship with many of the team members. In the event of a clinical risk event, the ward manager may need to caution or 'formally warn' the colleague he/she was socializing with the previous evening. If the colleague cannot differentiate between the role and the person, this can lead to many hurt feelings and confusion for both parties. This example also highlights one aspect of leadership that many find difficult—loneliness. However much a leader may wish to be part of the team, there will always need to be a degree of 'distancing' and of filtering of information known to the leader (because of his/her involvement at other levels within the organization) which it may not be possible or desirable to share with other team members. This usually becomes especially significant at times of organizational change, reviews of staffing levels, financial pressures, relocation of premises, closures and redundancies, etc. It can be very uncomfortable for the leader who is aware of the anxieties held by team members but not in a position to alleviate or give substance to those anxieties. The leader may also be accused of being unsupportive or withholding at a later stage when it becomes clear that the leader was party to information withheld from the team. While the reasons may be understood at a rational level, team members may still feel let down by a leader who 'could not trust them' to manage privileged information. It is important for this, and other reasons, that those in leadership positions establish some form of support or mentoring relationship outside of their work setting to help mitigate against the isolating aspects of leadership and provide a reflective, thinking, space in which the leader can process feelings and retain the capacity to think and be objective.

### Shared leadership

While leadership is often described as a role taken up by an individual, it may also be a quality possessed by many members of 'the team', even though only one person may be designated as such. Within the context of an interdisciplinary team, this becomes clear and relevant since the designated leadership role may move around and be 'taken up' by different people, according to the needs of the patient or the requirements of the task.

The close relationship between leadership and management has led the terms to be used interchangeably, but there is a difference in focus as Watson (1983) has indicated: managers tend toward a greater reliance on strategy, structure and systems, whereas leaders are more likely to focus on style, staff, skills and shared goals. However:

Increasingly, management and leadership are being seen as inextricably linked. It is one thing for a leader to propound a grand vision, but this is redundant unless the vision is managed so it becomes real achievement (Dearlove 2001, p. 538).

Within the setting of the NHS (UK), the old model which saw managers as those who planned and allocated resources while clinicians controlled and spent those resources can no longer be sustained. Transformational leadership, by which the leader influences staff (followers) for whom he/she is responsible by inspiring them with a vision of what can be achieved, is a favoured approach against a backdrop of an uncertain and turbulent work setting. A key proponent of this approach has been Bass (1994) who claims that transformational leadership enables the 'followers' to achieve far more than originally expected. For Bass, the effect of the leader on the followers is crucial and requires the leader to

- Generate greater awareness of the importance of the purpose of the organization and task outcomes
- Induce staff to transcend their own self-interests for the sake of the organization or team
- Activate the higher level needs of team members.

There are four basic components to transformational leadership:

- Idealized influence: which is reliant on the charisma of the leader and the respect and admiration of followers
- Inspirational motivation: where the leader's own behaviour provides meaning and challenge to the work.
- Intellectual stimulation: here the leader seeks from followers creative ways of resolving problems or novel ways of undertaking the work.
- Individualized consideration: the leader listens and has a clear concern for the growth and development needs of team members.

Within the NHS, the focus of leadership training is now changing to one where leaders (whether clinicians or managers) provide a strategic vision and leadership, with managers supporting them in the implementation and operationalization of that strategic vision. If the leadership is to be effective, then the role of 'follower' is clearly crucial. The key to leadership is in the ability to connect and interact with potential followers, most of whom want their leader to be genuine, have integrity and be worth following.

## Followership

Leaders require a degree of consent from members/followers that they are willing to be led, that they acknowledge the authority conferred upon the leader and accept that the leader has the right to implement decisions by exercising authority and power. As we shall discuss further in this chapter, leaders may choose to exert their authority to the full (by adopting an autocratic style) or may share their authority (by delegation) through the transfer of power, thus empowering others to act. There are limits to this in that the leader cannot transfer ultimate accountability for delivering the main task of the team, and this remains as a risk in delegatory leadership. If those to whom some authority and power has been delegated fail to succeed in what is required, the leader must still accept the responsibility for the negative outcome. The advice of Urwick, >50 years ago, still holds true. In his 10 principles of administration (or what we now term 'management'), he argues that authority should be commensurate with responsibility—the Principle of Correspondence (Urwick 1952). Hence, if you give someone a job to do, and are holding them accountable for its achievement, you must give them enough power to enable them to achieve what is required. Failure to do this will affect not only the outcome but also the motivation and leader–follower relationship.

Followership needs to be an active process of participation in the course of achieving the goals of the palliative care team. A core aspect of leadership, therefore, is to ensure that the concept of primary task is not only uppermost in the minds of members of the team, or organization, but is also constantly reviewed in the light of changing circumstances in the external environment, and that the team and organization adapt accordingly. This should be familiar to those engaged in palliative care where a similar approach is taken towards patient care: the alleviation of symptoms and enhancement of quality of life for the patient is uppermost in the minds of the palliative care team, and is constantly reviewed and adapted to by the team in the light of changing circumstances.

'Ownership' is an important factor in achieving satisfactory outcomes in that each team member needs to own a degree of responsibility for the overall life and work of the team. This ownership is wider than only engaging in issues which affects one's own personal comfort and work, or that of one's own immediate work group. It is tempting to split off and delegate, consciously and unconsciously, to senior management or the leader any sense of ownership and responsibility for the work, and overall good, of the organization as a whole. This implies that there must be some clear communication, at all levels of the organization, of both the vision and the strategy of the organization (e.g. NHS Trust Hospital, funding or charity) within which the team is located. It also follows that any strategic plan, business plan and operational policies formulated by the specialist palliative care team/unit should also relate clearly to those of the wider organization. Staff appraisal, job profiles and individual training plans should also inter-relate with the wider organization. The leader will be the most likely person to interface with other aspects of the organization, but he/she needs to ensure there is genuine consultation, participation and involvement in the development of these different documents if followers are to believe they are a valued part of the process of shaping the service as well as its delivery. This also has relevance for 'user' involvement if users are to take some ownership, through partnership, of the health outcome and treatment process (see later and Chapter 4 of this volume). By using the word 'process', I am implying that time is required for this activity. Decisions have to be taken as to how much time should be spent on consultation and participation in decision making by members. Some members may wish to be more actively involved than others. However, all should have some degree of ownership in the aims of the team and in providing a quality service to patients, as well as supporting each other in achieving that. Much of this work can be a part of a wider focus on team building (see Chapter 8 of this volume), whether as part of a weekly meeting or a specially designated 'away day' when some of these issues can be addressed without the same pressure of immediate patient need, telephone and pager demands. As mentioned above, various members/followers may also have leadership qualities and skills, and it is important, especially in multi- and interdisciplinary teamwork, that they are willing to take on any leadership role available to them. This can allow their creative and managerial skills to develop, as well as provide insight into the hardships and vicissitudes of management and leadership, together with an appreciation of the loneliness inherent in the role.

The issue of readiness to follow has been addressed by Hersey and Blanchard (1993) who describe readiness, not as a personal characteristic, but as the extent to which followers have the ability and willingness to accomplish a specific task. From this, they derive a continuum of four levels of readiness (R1 low follower readiness–R4 high follower readiness). For each level, they suggest there is an appropriate leadership style (S1–S4) which blends 'task behaviour' with 'relationship behaviour':

- S1 *Telling* Emphasizes high amounts of guidance (task behaviour) but limited support (relationship behaviour). Most appropriate style for low follower readiness (R1)
- S2 *Selling* High amount of both directive (task) and relationship behaviour. More appropriate to low to moderate follower behaviour (R2)
- S3 *Participating* High amounts of two-way communication and supportive (relationship) behaviour, but low amount of guidance (task). Especially applicable for moderate to high follower readiness (R3)
- S4 *Delegating* Little direction, or support, provided hence low levels of both task and relationship behaviours. This style is best suited to those exhibiting high follower readiness (R4)

The main relevance of this model is that it focuses our attention on developing, to the extent to which they are willing to go, the ability, confidence and commitment of colleagues. It also implies a need for the leader to 'titrate' the amounts of task and relationship behaviour in order to balance direction and support with motivation. This has clear implications beyond leadership to the wider issues of training and team development (see Chapters 8 and 10 of this volume).

## Distributive leadership

One aspect of leadership and followership which has been explored in recent years is that of 'collective' or 'distributed' leadership. Huffington *et al.* (2004) describe how many organizations are seeking to have 'flatter' structures, with more inter- and cross-functional teams often forming alliances with customers and competitors. 'Decisions need to be taken away from the centre of the organization, at the point of contact between the organization and its environment' (Huffington *et al.* 2004, p. 68). Within palliative care, especially home care, this will be familiar in that a team member visiting a patient at home may need to make changes to the care plan in the light of a change in the condition of the patient or the family. These decisions may be made in collaboration with non-specialist palliative care team members (such as community nurses or family doctors). It may or may not be possible to contact other team members immediately to consult about the decision. If not, the team member in the home would need to have sufficient authority to make whatever decision was necessary at the time in the best interests of the patient. Subsequently that decision would usually be fed back to other members of the palliative care team and either be ratified or changed following discussion, with maintenance of continuity of patient care being a prime concern.

Distributive leadership, while empowering the individual, does not remove accountability, and this can result in a sense of vulnerability through enhancing individual responsibility to report back, to be monitored and receive feedback from others on decisions made. Such situations also raise issues, for the palliative team member, regarding their own confidence in their role and experience when working alongside other professional colleagues of a different discipline. The ability to manage oneself in a role and contain any anxiety and uncertainty regarding relationships with other disciplines is of great significance. Failure to manage this is often a contributory factor in the antagonistic or recriminatory actions which sometimes arise in multiprofessional relationships. If these tensions are not resolved satisfactorily, the individual can experience intense vulnerability, respond at a purely visceral emotional level and lose the capacity to think. It is important that the leader creates a 'containing' structure conducive to creativity and thought. Failure, by the leader, to provide such emotional containment and boundary management can be a contributory factor in the individual feeling 'abandoned' by the team or organization. This isolation can then lead to the experience of feeling bullied by those (often of other disciplines) who are questioning both the decisions and the right to make those decisions. It is as if those to whom authority has been delegated experience themselves as wholly accountable and needing to support or authorize each other laterally because the senior management, or leadership, has abdicated its role and abandoned the team member to 'fend for themselves'.

In thinking about the application of these ideas to specialist palliative care, it is interesting to look at the experience of a group of assistant directors of local authority services exercising leadership horizontally in a partnership of peer organizations, all of whom may be looking for a leadership role. Huffington *et al.* describe a workshop in which the assistant directors explored the issues:

The assistant directors identified that their traditional way of working was to work solo in expert roles in which they could demonstrate individual competence. In working across organizational boundaries they discovered that expertise must be exchanged and colleagues would need to work together seamlessly to deliver a satisfactory outcome. This meant that individual competence did not have to be demonstrated in the same way. It would need to be combined with the skills of creating personal relationships with strategic partners, and expertise needed to be seen as the material that could be shared, bartered, and consulted. This meant that the leadership development of these assistant directors had to focus on personal development, group working, and influencing skills in which they would learn to lead from an awareness of personal values and principles and learn skills in collaborative working. Simultaneously, they would need to be able to balance and resolve any issues deriving from the constant need for systems of account-ability and responsibility. It was as if they had to blend hierarchical and horizontal leadership together so as to weave the weft and warp of a new organizational fabric (Huffington *et al.* 2004, p. 76).

This account would seem to reflect the evolutionary or developmental process within many teams as they move across the spectrum from multidisciplinary to interdisciplinary working. The interdisciplinary team within specialist pal-liative care will contain people who are very competent in their own profes-sion and aware of the expertise they bring to the work of the team. However, it may be challenging to be accountable, or responsible, to a leader of a different discipline who seeks to examine the reasoning behind decisions made, or a colleague's failure to 'report back', etc. It can be even more difficult if the questions are being asked by other team members not in a designated leader-ship role. As mentioned in Chapter 2, there needs to be a high degree of trust, respect and confidence in each other's role and competence if such question-ing and explanation is to remain creative and 'on task' and not be experienced as persecutory or demeaning of one's role and contribution.

If this trustful, creative and emotionally 'containing' environment can be established, then each individual can retain their own competence and authority. They will also be better able to learn from others, and contribute to the learning of others within the team.

## Authority

Authority refers to the right to make ultimate decisions and legitimizes the capability to exercise influence over the behaviour, priorities and activities of others. Responsibility and accountability normally come with authority, espe-cially in relation to the results achieved by given activities. Authority describes a relationship which is recognized by those concerned and involves exertion on the part of the leader and acceptance by the follower, so that there is a degree of common consent of the authority exercised on behalf of the organ-ization and expressed through the role one occupies. In a fairly hierarchical setting, this can be clearly understood. However, in many palliative care settings, this may not be so clear as there are often multiple 'stakeholders' who may lay claim to ownership—charitable funding bodies, users, strategic health authority, primary care team, staff, professional groups, unions, etc. These different groups may have varied opinions as to where authority comes from, to whom it is delegated and to what extent, all of which could influence the decision-making ability of the leader. (See Chapter 12)

When team members take up a follower role within the team, they are, at least implicitly, delegating some of their personal authority to the person in the leadership role. If there is ambivalence about the leader, then the follower may sanction the authority of the role, but not of the person in the role. This means that there is a potential risk of sabotaging or undermining of the leader when he or she seeks to act authoritatively. Most leaders would acknowledge to themselves, if not publicly, that there are always limits to the authority they have, and of the need to monitor the conscious and unconscious forces within the team that enhance or diminish the leader's authority.

In the course of our own personal growth and development, we will have experienced a variety of authority figures within our family, society, our schooling and our work life. Some of these we will have internalized as 'in-the-mind' authority figures which will have varying powers to affect us in later life—even after they have died. For example, if we have been told by past authority figures that we are 'stupid' or 'always indecisive', this can lead to much self-doubt and lack of confidence in later life. In terms of leadership and authority, this can lead to the individual finding it difficult to believe in themselves in a leadership role, and in their competence to take up authority even when clearly sanctioned by others. There can be a constant fear that 'one day I will be found out as a fraud'. The influence of one's inner-world need not undermine our ability to function effectively in a role provided we have some degree of understanding and recognition of those aspects of our role that we sometimes find difficult.

The opposite end of the spectrum is represented by those whose inner-world figures seem to give them a sense of omnipotence, one who can do no wrong. In certain professions, such people can become arrogant and pompous, with little capacity to listen to or learn from others, and frequently it is very difficult for others to work with or be clients or patients of such people. They rapidly progress from being authoritative to being authoritarian, with damaging effects on those around.

## Power

Power, in contrast to authority, is an attribute of the person not the role, and is a capability that arises from both internal and external sources. Some view power as a resource possessed by certain individuals or groups. Others see it in terms of a social relationship characterized by some form of dependency, relating to the ability to control or influence the behaviour of others, with or without their consent.

- Externally, power comes from what the person controls, which may be money, a reference, promotion prospects or the ability to provide a car park space.
- Internally, power comes from the individual's knowledge, experience, how they present themselves and therefore their self-image, the strength of their personality.

What is of greater importance than actual power is the perceived power that others believe the leader or other person to possess. This links to Robbins (1998) who suggests that as power may exist but not be used it implies a potential that need not be actualized to be effective. Power is therefore a capacity or a potential. 'A person can have power over you only if he or she controls something you desire' (Robbins 1998, p. 396). Similarly, Morgan sees power as the 'medium through which conflicts of interest are ultimately resolved. Power influences who gets what, when and how' (Morgan 1986, p. 158). It is important always to remember that we are dealing with organizations that exist through human relationships and there can therefore only ever be partial control over the work behaviour of others. More is achieved through the processes of negotiation, persuasion and manipulation than through systems of rules and official procedures (Watson 2002).

The sources of power are rich and varied, and Morgan (1986, p. 159) provides a wide list, many of which begin with the word 'control': control of scarce resource, control of knowledge and information, of decision processes, of technology, etc. as well as personal ability such as the ability to cope with uncertainty, as well the power one already has. Morgan sees these sources of power as providing members of organizations with a variety of means for enhancing their interests and resolving or perpetuating conflict.

French and Raven (1986) have identified five main sources of power in organizations:

- **Reward power**—the use of rewards to influence people, especially if those rewards are desired by the target group.
- **Coercive power**—this can be a crude use of power to threaten or punish (often by sanctions or threats of dismissal) in order to achieve a goal.
- **Legitimate power**—derives from the person's position in the organization and links with an understanding of authority as the power to act.
- **Referrant power**—this is concerned with personal power and is generally understood as 'charisma'. It is often dependent upon the perception and recognition by other people. As such, it can dissipate and be lost, such as when the charismatic leader may no longer be needed once a particular crisis has ended.

- **Expert power**—this usually derives from possessing specialist knowledge and skills. However, it is also dependent on others recognizing and valuing that expertise, thus giving it credibility.

These different sources of power can be easily identified in most organizations and may emerge in the life of a multi- or interdisciplinary team at various points in its history. The way in which the leadership addresses the primary task and utilizes power will be influential in both the life of the team and the relationship with patients and families. 'Expertise' is almost built into a specialist team, and each team member will have specialist knowledge and skill to contribute to the overall life and work of the team. How such expertise is shared within the team and with other professionals will be influential in terms of inter- and intrateam dynamics. However, while the contribution of expert knowledge is usually valued, in recent years such expertise has been challenged by some 'users' of services who wish to contribute their knowledge and experience to the planning and provision of services (see Chapter 4 of this volume). This can be a factor in the provision of care to patients with chronic conditions and is likely to be especially relevant as palliative care widens its remit to non-cancer conditions.

For example, Sue was a middle aged lady with disseminated sclerosis. On one occasion she was admitted to hospital, at a time when her usual consultant was away, and was seen by a new junior doctor. He examined Sue and announced that her medication was all wrong and he was going to change it and 'sort her out'. In response to her question 'What are you proposing?' he outlined the radical changes he was going to make. Sue knew from previous experience that his proposed changes would exacerbate her condition and reduce her quality of life. She had been down this pathway before with his predecessor. What she needed initially was some respite care. The doctor was unable or unwilling to listen to her, or her experience of living with this illness. The ward sister/manager intervened and supported Sue's viewpoint.

The dynamic between the patient and the doctor epitomized a classic 'power–powerlessness' tension whereby the patient is assigned the role of being the compliant, passive recipient of a care plan developed by others as 'experts'. However, many patients now wish to participate far more in the care planning and wish for their views and experience of the illness to be heard and valued. User involvement, in all its different forms, can be challenging of the power of the professional who may need to surrender some of that power if a true partnership is to develop.

## Empowerment

Empowerment is usually understood in terms of empowering staff by delegating to the most appropriate level of responsibility. However, as has been indicated above, it may be seen in terms of users as well as staff. In the world of management, Peters (1988) says that 'Empowerment really boils down to "taking seriously". No one denies where the answers are: on the firing line. How do we get people to come forth and give answers, to take risks by trying new things . . . ?' He suggests that the answer is to listen to staff, defer to the front line, delegate and install a horizontal style of management. For team leaders, the application of this to the leader–follower relationship is clear, but what of the users of the service?

If we think of the provision of palliative care, it would seem to imply: listen to the patient, defer to their experience of living with the disease and incorporate the patient into the decision-making process. Providing patients and families with clearly understood information about their illness and treatment, in a sensitive and appropriate manner, is central in good care. The consultation should also be purposeful and real if the patient is to believe that their opinion and feelings are valued. For empowerment to happen, it is necessary for those in authority to be able to 'let go' sufficiently to allow real sharing to occur.

Monroe and Oliviere (2003, p. 140) indicate that 'involving patients in their care is fundamental in palliative care and is linked to enhancement of human dignity, increased patient satisfaction, a greater efficacy of health education and improved compliance'. They highlight that, for patient partnership and choices to be real, several things need to be in place: knowledge of what is available in terms of treatment and palliative care, staff being able to communicate effectively and sensitively, and staff having a supportive environment if they are to be able to engage in sensitive conversations. The staff also need to have an open attitude to exploring need and restoring a degree of control and choice to the patient/family. While patients and families may have access to a great deal of information via the Internet and a variety of self-help groups, they may not have the capacity to sift that information and know what weight to give to the various opinions and advice given within those sources. Rather than patients feeling threatened by staff, there are times when the staff may feel threatened by patients who come 'armed' with large print-outs of information about their disease and treatment/care options culled from the Internet. However, the inability of patients to evaluate the information properly may, in effect, render them powerless rather than powerful as a result of their searches. The key issue, once again, is the establishment of a relationship of openness and trust between professional caregiver and patient if the effects of the power–powerless dynamic are not to dominate and spoil the relationship and the quality of care given and received.

In respect of staff, empowerment means making people responsible for the quality of their own work and providing them with the means to test it is working by ensuring they receive direct feedback from the 'customer, client, patient'. Leaders and managers therefore need to adopt a consultative style of working and listen to the views of their staff, especially when change is being contemplated. The main benefits of empowerment are that the organization and team can make maximum use of the knowledge held by the various members to enhance the service provided. Empowerment also leads to greater 'ownership' of the results of any change programme and is especially important when there is a high degree of uncertainty within the organization in which the team is located.

Empowerment is very much concerned with values and the belief that people matter, because they are people more than a resource or a cost for the organization. Communication and trust are major factors in empowerment, and team working is a fundamental requirement if empowerment is to be effective. There has to be a genuine sharing of information, views and rewards between members, whether the team has a permanent membership or a more temporary structure as in a project team. Empowerment brings a shift in emphasis, in that status comes more from the skills and knowledge held than from power and position within the team or organization. Evaluating whether empowerment enhances effectiveness is difficult but important. In fact, determining whether team working is effective is also very difficult. Performance measures may be easier within a manufacturing industry, in that one can measure output, cost, profit, downtime and quality. However, this is not so easy in a health care environment, though measuring activity levels does happen. More human measures also exist in that one can monitor sickness absence (especially stress-related), attitudes, satisfaction, etc. However, obtaining an objective measure of some of these factors can be more difficult and does not always provide meaningful results. Much work is needed towards finding appropriate and satisfactory ways of determining whether or not a team has effective leadership and is working effectively towards achieving its primary purpose. We can count the number of visits made by a caregiver to a number of patients, but how do we know the quality of interaction between a particular caregiver and an individual patient. Is the subjective satisfaction level reported by the patient sufficient? (see Chapter 13 of this volume).

## Bullying and harassment

### Within teams and organizations

It is important to maintain a watch over the ways in which power and authority are used within both the organization and the team to ensure they continue to be used legitimately and fairly. Power can be misused and often shows itself in terms of the following

## FAVOURITISM

This may be real or as perceived by others. A leader may be thought to have a favourite. If this is a fact, it can quickly become divisive in a team; if it is not true, then it may indicate envy and rivalry between some team members which may be operating at an unconscious level and, therefore, not be overt and easily identified. Favouritism also represents a failure to maintain an equal opportunities stance, and may be at variance with the mission statement and policies of the organization. If, for example, a team leader develops a culture of team members going to a local pub for a drink at the end of the day, this can discriminate against those who have family commitments or do not like pubs. If the discussion is work related with opinions shared and decisions made, those not present can feel, and are, excluded from what can be perceived as the 'in-crowd'. Those who feel excluded can be under great pressure to conform by attending or run the risk of being disadvantaged.

## VICTIMIZATION

This can be claimed when another's prospects are blocked or restricted. This may also lead to scapegoating if there is a need to find someone to blame, often for the leader's errors or ineffectiveness.

## LACK OF MANNERS AND RESPECT

Speaking rudely to others and humiliating staff in public may be a displacement reaction of feelings aroused by a confrontational carer–patient interaction. If the patient has been abusive and the carer or caregiver does not wish to retaliate with rudeness, the next non-patient who confronts the carer or makes demands may be responded to with 'uncharacteristic' rudeness. This unconscious behaviour needs to be identified and addressed in the context of the team dynamic at an appropriate team meeting. However, treating others with contempt by demeaning them in public is a different matter. Disciplining a staff member in public shows lack of respect for the person being disciplined and humiliated in this way. It can also have an effect on those who witness such behaviour.

Harassment and bullying may take several different forms on grounds of race, gender, religion, disability, or personal likes and dislikes.

For example, John was a deputy director who worked with Anthea, the Director of Patient Services. John worked hard, was very competent in his previous job, but no longer felt able to meet the expectations of his new boss. He was often only given a partial briefing for required reports and documents. Often it was evident that Anthea was not clear what she wanted and only clarified the brief once John's fourth or fifth draft was in the shredder. John's effectiveness started to diminish over time. To get to Anthea's office, he had to walk through the typing pool and he became increasingly nervous of team meetings as Anthea would point out his inadequacies before his colleagues. On several occasions, during a one-to-one meeting she would reduce him to tears and then terminate the meetings, opening the office door and ushering him out into the typing pool. Here he would have to walk through the office, obviously distressed, and feeling totally humiliated and emasculated.

Harassment and bullying not only cause strain to relationships at work but can also affect home life. Over time, the person who is being harassed will lose their motivation to work, depending on how incidents are dealt with. They will also lose respect for their managers and their colleagues, especially if it is felt that colleagues are unable, or unprepared, to speak out about incidents of bullying behaviour they have witnesed. Victims of workplace bullying talk of experiencing insomnia, depression, nervousness, apathy and lack of concentration, and some may attempt or actually commit suicide.

The bullying behaviour may not be physical but may include ridicule, public humiliation (as in the above example) and verbal threats. There may also be deliberate social isolation and changes of work tasks and expectations which can result in increased difficulty in successfully completing what is expected. In some organizations or work groups, such events form part of the culture, with further ridicule if the individual cannot 'cope' with teasing and insults. Where the whole group becomes involved, it becomes easier for the behaviour to persist as any guilt that might otherwise be felt is dissipated amongst the group members. If the victims complain, their complaint tends to disturb the equilibrium of the organization and so may be 'played down' by senior managers, with labelling of the victim as a 'wimp' or a 'difficult colleague'. It is not always a junior being bullied by a senior since the behaviour may be within the peer group. It can also be from a subordinate to a senior, as in the case of an individual who seeks to 'manipulate' the leader in order to meet their own needs over those of the team. Sometimes, rather than person–person bullying, it is the organization itself that is the 'bully'. In such cases, harassment or bullying can be experienced as a result of the way in which statistics are used to highlight the failure of individuals to meet targets (waiting times, number of visits made, number of patients seen, number of days of in-patient care, financial targets, etc.). It is not that such targets may not be important, but the way in which they are used by the organization or stakeholders which can be experienced as punitive, oppressive and a major source of work-related stress.

It is important that any organization and team has a robust approach to bullying and harassment, backed up by policies and access to a confidential route to report such behaviour with appropriate support for victims. Those who take up a leadership role have a responsibility to monitor the ways in which power is used by themselves and by others in their relationships at work, with each other and with their clients.

## Abusive patients and families

In discussing harassment and bullying within the organization and within teams, it is important to acknowledge that it may be the client or their family who seek to bully and harass staff. Within palliative care, most of the patients have a life-threatening condition, but this does not give them the freedom to abuse the staff who offer care. A degree of regression can occur for some patients who, in effect, may have a childlike tantrum because what they want is not being provided immediately. It is sometimes difficult for staff to establish clear boundaries because they become subverted by the fact that this person is dying and staff should be understanding and nice at all times. However, as with young children, regressed adults can feel frightened by their rage and violent outbursts. The rage may be directed at the staff or at the family, and they may fear going completely out of control. It can be important for staff to re-state or re-establish boundaries of non-acceptable behaviour. The patient can feel safer and more secure knowing that the staff are not going to abandon them because of their outburst, but are capable of 'containing' the emotion and managing the boundaries for them. Staff who experience such interactions also need to know that they have the active support of their colleagues. It is now common in many hospitals for there to be notices stating that the Trust Hospital will take firm action, and may prosecute, anyone who abuses staff in any way. In addition, staff need to know that the Trust will indeed act and that there will be appropriate support for any staff member who is abused by clients during their time at work.

## Conclusion

Within the context of specialist palliative care, a variety of types of team exist. In some teams, leadership may be vested in one named individual and remain there. If, however, the team moves towards a more interdisciplinary model, there may be more sharing of the leadership with other team members depending on the needs of the patient and family, or the skills needed to fulfil a particular task. Leadership may thus move around within the team. The use, and abuse, of power and authority is a key issue for anyone in leadership and should be one of the areas focused upon as part of the ongoing reflective practice of all team members. Empowering staff and users of the service will always have implications for the well-being of all team members and the dynamic they create.

# References

Bass BM and Avolio BJ (1994). *Improving Organizational Performance Through Transformational Leadership*. Sage Publications, London.

Dearlove D (2001). Reinventing leadership. In: Crainer S and Dearlove D, ed. *Financial Times Handbook of Management*, 2nd edn. Financial Times-Prentice Hall, Harlow, UK, p. 538.

French JP and Raven B (1986). The bases of social power. In: Cartwright D and Zander AE, ed. *Group Dynamics: Research and Theory*, 3rd edn. Harper and Row, Beaconsfield, UK, pp. 150–167.

Hersey P and Blanchard KH (1993). *Management of Organizational Behaviour: Utilizing Human Resources*, 6th edn. Prentice Hall, Harlow, UK.

Huffington C, James K and Armstrong D (2004). What is the emotional cost of distributed leadership? In: Huffington C, Armstrong D, Halton W, Hoyle L and Pooley J., ed. *Working Below the Surface: The Emotional Life of Contemporary Organizations*. Karnac, London, pp. 67–84.

Levine S and Crom M (1994). *The Leader in You*. Simon and Schuster, London.

Monroe B and Oliviere D, eds. (2003) *Patient Participation in Palliative Care: A Voice for the Voiceless*. Oxford University Press, Oxford.

Morgan G (1986). *Images of Organization*. Sage Publications, London.

Peters T (1988). *Thriving on Chaos*. MacMillan, Basingstoke, UK.

Robbins SP (1998). *Organizational Behaviour*, 8th edn. Prentice-Hall, Harlow, UK, p. 396.

Urwick L (1952). *The Elements of Administration*. Pitman, London.

Watson CM (1983). Leadership, management and the seven keys. *Business Horizons* March–April, 8–13.

Watson TJ (2002). *Organising and Managing Work: Organisational, Managerial and Strategic Behaviour in Theory and Practice*. Financial Times Prentice-Hall, Harlow, UK.

# 6

# Sitting close to death

*Noreen Ramsay*

[*Editors comment*: when your daily work takes you constantly to the sharp edge of human suffering it is often difficult to see and reflect accurately on all that is happening at the interface between patients, carers and the health care professionals offering care. Those who work in such settings will be aware of the way in which the suffering seen and experienced at work can be mirrored in suffering and anxiety experienced by the staff. Within organizations such as health care, we are familiar with the way in which we develop defences to protect ourselves against a level of anxiety that could disable us and render us unable to function in our work role. If the leadership and management is able to provide sufficient containment for anxiety, this can have a very positive effect on the workers and on job satisfaction. One way of identifying what happens at the interface between patient and professional caregiver is to undertake an observation over time. The method of observing an organization, such as a palliative care unit, is described by Hinshelwood and Skogstad (2000). They advocate the use of a psychoanalytical participant observation which has five aspects:

- A way of observing with 'evenly hovering attention' and without premature judgement
- Careful use of the observer's subjective experience
- The capacity to reflect and think about the experience as a whole
- The recognition of the unconscious dimension
- The formulation of interpretations which provide a means of verifying (or falsifying) the conclusions the analyst has reached through this process.

The observation study is supplemented by supervisory seminars which can help the observer to observe his/her own experiences within the culture of the ward, unit or organization. In this way, the observer picks up the 'atmosphere', and the application of this lies in sensitizing to the dynamic of the setting and helping people move nearer to being observing participants within their work setting.

The following chapter describes an observation of a palliative care unit and the effect of undertaking this study on the individual observer. For myself, it mirrors my own experiences of a similar observation study undertaken >30 years ago on a psycho-geriatric admission ward (Speck 1970). Such studies can be uncomfortable for the observer but do provide us with a very valuable insight into the effects of the work undertaken in health care on the staff group. The chapter (Ramsay 2000) is therefore reproduced, with permission, as a way of helping us reflect and identify some of the interactions that can be experienced within palliative care [P. Speck].

# Sitting close to death: A palliative care unit

*Noreen Ramsay*

## Introduction

Death is as natural a phenomenon as birth. Our society has become distanced from both. Increasingly death, like birth, has been taken over by medical specialists and removed from its place within the natural cycle of the family. This creates difficulties for the individual undergoing the private, personal experience of the process of dying within a medical setting. It also creates difficulties and challenges for those professionals caring for them. In the last 20 years the development of the Hospice movement came with a recognition that hospitals concerned with giving acute medical care did not enable people to die with dignity and respect. In hospitals with a primarily diagnostic and curative attitude, dying was seen as a failure. Palliative care developed as a patient centred approach to physical, psychological and spiritual healing, its primary aim being the relief of distressing symptoms in order to allow the person to make the best possible use of whatever life they have left, potentially enabling the process of dying to be one of personal growth (Saunders 1960). I was initially attracted as a junior doctor to the ideas of the hospice philosophy because of their recognition of the impact of patient care on the professionals working with the dying patient. This understanding was blatantly lacking in my experience of acute general medicine.

With the recognition of palliative medicine as a speciality in medicine and the rapid growth of services for the dying in the health service, a growing number of professionals are involved with the dying. Working so closely with the reality of death stirs up anxieties that need to be defended against, in order not to be overwhelmed by them. These defences may be helpful in enabling professionals to continue to offer something useful to dying patients. The palliative care unit as a whole will develop its own defensive system in order to reduce the level of anxiety of those working there. Like all defences, this system may be helpful, but may also develop in such a way as to hinder the primary task of patient care. Menzies ([1959] 1988) described a similar process in a paper which looks at the development of nursing practices. The influence of defensive dynamics on the working practices of a unit are not always recognised.

## The ward observation

As a psychiatrist I became involved in liaison work in a hospice and worked with medical teams in the care of patients dying with Aids. While I knew I had an interest in this area, I was apprehensive about pursuing it further without being able to answer questions about its personal impact. It is difficult to answer these questions while one is busy in a unit, taking an active part in the dynamics of the situation oneself.

I thought that the opportunity to do a ward observation of a palliative care unit would enable me to observe the functioning of the unit. In fact, I became more aware of my own defences. The palliative care unit I observed was in a separate building on the site of a district general hospital. The main work of the team was community based and therefore not accessible to me. The 25 in-patient beds were used for terminal care, assessment and relief of intractable symptoms and respite care. The unit was primarily nursing-led with lesser input from medical staff. It had been in existence for about eight years.

The ward observation was structured so that I sat in the corridor of the unit, in the same place, at the same time, for one hour a week, over 12 weeks. I wrote up my observations afterwards and discussed them in a fortnightly supervision. The method of observing and the function of such a seminar are described in more detail in Hinshelwood and Skogstad (2000).

## Isolated by privacy

In the first few observation sessions my initial impression was of isolation. This was emphasised externally by the concrete structures. The unit was separate from the main building of the general hospital. It was not easy to walk between the two. I was told the building was originally designed as an isolation unit, only later being taken over as a hospice. For security reasons the front door was locked, a buzzer system being used to gain admittance. The effect of this arrangement was that those with terminal illness, while in the same grounds as the general hospital, were effectively isolated from it.

Within the unit itself the emphasis was on privacy. The majority of the patients' rooms were private single rooms, with the only double rooms being occupied by patients who were not actually dying. Many of the doors were shut or left ajar. Each door had a notice which either said 'Do not disturb' or 'Knock before entering'. During a period when some of the patients were being barrier-nursed because of infection, this was changed to 'Do not enter, ask a staff member before entering'.

The only public area, the communal day room, was remarkable in its lack of use. Patients used it mainly to speak on the telephone, and staff used it for formal meetings. The only patient who seemed to inhabit this area regularly was an elderly lady who stood out from the other patients because of her air of independence and liveliness as she pushed herself around in her wheelchair. New patients, unsure of their place in the unit, made brief exploratory excursions into the corridor or day room, and then retreated to their rooms. The kitchen area was used mainly by relatives to do practical tasks such as making tea or washing up cups.

As an observer seated in the corridor I was aware of my position in the public space, which was at times dead quiet. All the life and all the dying was going on in the rooms, which were closed off and inaccessible to me.

On my introduction to the unit I was shown all around the building and introduced to many of the staff and the unit cat. I was not shown a patient's room and did not meet any patient – 'for obvious reasons', I was told. Even the nursing staff hesitated to enter those rooms without some form of permission. They responded to a request for help from a patient by answering a 'call light' very quickly, but still knocked before entering the room. They glanced into rooms as they went along the corridor, or peered through the shutters on the door windows without opening a closed door and did not enter unless help was obviously needed. Volunteers were similarly tentative when offering their services. My own experience of this respectful distance and unwillingness to intrude was that the few people who approached me usually made a tentative enquiry as to whether I was waiting for someone or whether I wanted any tea. When I declined these offers there was no follow-up to my response and I was left alone. Despite an external appearance of openness and friendliness, there was the impression that something was being kept firmly locked away.

## Faced with the horror of death

Over the next three sessions I saw glimpses of the reality around me which I had felt isolated from. These images made me wonder what was going on in this place. The homely furnishings, mixed with hospital tea trolleys and oxygen cylinders, gave an appearance of the trappings of a friendly hospital with its routines and hierarchy of staff, busy going about their duties. Gradually I felt exposed to something much greater, more primitive and uncontrollable, in the face of which I was helpless.

### Session 3

*Throughout the earlier part of the session a baby was crying in one of the rooms and I sat wondering why the baby was there, why its mother was there and what was on her mind.*

*Towards the end, a family started to come out of one of the rooms further down the corridor and I thought I might be able to answer my questions, as they started to walk towards me. I was struck by a stiffness and formality in the way they all moved, particularly in the little boy of about four who seemed uncomfortable with his role of leading them down the corridor. It was more like a funeral procession than a walk to the day room to look for some toys to play with. Behind him was a woman in an electric wheelchair, whose young face and body were blown up to a grotesque size by the side-effects of steroids. Her legs dangled huge with swelling. She moved beside the pushchair where the baby wriggled in protest. A woman of similar age pushed the baby. She was thin, her face drawn taut, her body stiffly held upright. An older woman walked behind them, more at ease than the others.*

*They passed by me into the day room, making brief eye contact with me, asking the boy if he remembered where the toys were kept. They only stayed a few minutes, standing around awkwardly. The thin woman suggested they go somewhere else, a conservatory, where there would be toys and beanbags for the children. As they started to leave the unit, one of the nurses protested that the patient would freeze if she went out and insisted on getting a cardigan for her. They all waited stiffly in the corridor while the nurse got a rug for her shoulders and went back for another for her legs.*

*As I left the unit at the end of that session I glimpsed a man lying in bed. He saw me as I went by and raised himself onto one thin elbow and stretched out the other arm to me. 'Nurse', he called, eyes staring from his skull. I walked on and fled from my helplessness. During the week I was haunted by the images of his emaciated face, raised to me, and of the family walking down the corridor towards me.*

### Session 4

*In the room nearest to me, a woman's voice was raised in response to gentle enquiries from her husband and son. She repeated 'yes, yes, yes, yes' in a loud monotonous tone to each enquiry. Not fully conscious, she struggled to maintain contact with them. Throughout the whole hour I listened to her voice.*

*A young man left the day room where he had been talking to an older couple and went into one of the rooms. Shortly afterwards he re-emerged with a young woman and they walked side by side, very slowly towards the day room. They paused to smile and comment on the damage done to the wallpaper by the cat. Her face rounded by steroids was still pretty and she was about the same age as I was. She glanced at me as she passed, but I could not maintain eye contact. I was too overwhelmed by the large ugly scar over her scalp, not yet concealed, where the hair was growing back on her shaven head.*

*An alarm call from one of the rooms sounded. No one responded. I sat and listened to it, becoming more and more anxious, wanting someone to do something, but feeling unable to act myself. It rang for several minutes.*

*Session 5*

*The night before the observation I had a dream about being in the unit. In this dream, I was in the corridor near to where I usually sat, but I was lying on the floor, being held up by my arms and feet by two nurses. My body was floppy and my limbs hung useless as a rag doll's as they tried to drag me along the floor. The feeling was of complete helplessness. Following this dream, I was apprehensive about what experience I was to be subjected to during this session.*

*I met the unit's black cat outside. This was unusual. Also unusual was that instead of his normally self-contained and independent attitude he came over to me looking to be stroked. I helped him to come through the door. The receptionist told me that he had been in and out about four times that afternoon and did not seem to know where he wanted to be. She said, 'We lost one today, he always senses it.' On the way down the corridor I passed an empty room with the bed made up and presumed this was the room where someone had died that day. There was an initial air of business on the unit, with people coming and going to the rooms. For the first time the fire doors were open in the day room. I was aware of a thin young Indian man sitting behind me in the day room reading a book and watching the corridor. Then one of the nurses started closing the room doors and the shutters on the door windows in a brisk business-like fashion until all the corridor was sealed off. Only myself and the man behind me remained watching. The receptionist opened the doors at the other end and stood there, while the nurse remained in the middle of the corridor, both on guard. Two men in white coats wheeled a metal box on a trolley into one of the rooms and shortly afterwards came out and wheeled it off the unit. I felt for the other watcher. What must it be like to see this while sitting in vigil for a dying relative? The receptionist left her post and the nurse relaxed as she slowly went about the ward opening doors and windows. Gradually life returned to the ward. The nurses retreated into the staff room and discussed women's rights, etiquette and feminism. I sat, not quite able to believe what had happened.*

The shuttering off of the ward was strongly reminiscent of the closing of curtains around beds on large wards when someone has died in a general hospital. It seemed an anxious attempt to shutter off from the reality of the death of a human being. The lack of acknowledgement left me isolated and wishing for the comfort of one of those cups of tea they were always offering. The only creature that expressed distress was the cat. One of the volunteers said she would go and let him in as he was howling outside. Later he went into one of the empty rooms and started ripping up the carpet with his claws. This place felt frightening. Beneath the veneer of a hospital it was a place where rituals were carried out involving the passage towards death, and the cat knew about it. There was something much older and more powerful, in the face of which modern medicine and my professional training were impotent – as I had been in my dream.

## Exposed alone

In the following week, I felt both anger and pain. The anger was at what I perceived to be a superficial response to another's suffering and the pain was for the isolation of a man dying alone.

### Session 6

*An older woman, small beside a tall grey-haired younger man, walked towards me, his arm around her shoulder.*

'How are you doing, Amy?'

*Somewhat hesitantly, her voice croaking, she said 'I'm doing all right.'*

'You seem stronger today.' *She did not look sure about this.* 'Does Jack recognise you today?', *he asked as they went past me.*

*The conversation continued, partly audible in the corridor while they made tea in the kitchen, her voice low and sad, while he spoke in a loud cheerful manner.*

'It makes you think about mercy killing, but the doctors don't agree with it,' *he said.*

'While there's life there is still hope,' *she replied.*

'Not at this stage,' *he answered.*

'When you are married that long, they are part of your life.'

'I don't know, I've not been married that long.'

'He's 84.'

'We all have to go sometime.'

*She said,* 'Life goes on, but it's never the same again, you never get over it.'

'It depends what you mean get over it. When my father died I was really upset, but I had my life to live, I just got on with it.'

'When you are together 40 years they are part of you', *she said.*

'Did you meet Mrs S? Her husband died last week, very suddenly.'

*'It's better like that,' she replied.*

*'Oh no, you don't have any warning, you feel cheated.'*

*'It's the monotony of just sitting there.'*

*'You don't want either really, do you? You are not used to it. You have never seen someone like this before? Your parents, when they died what age were they?'*

*'My mother was 69.'*

*'Did she collapse suddenly or get thin and die slowly?'*

As I listened to the stream of clichés, discussing such major issues loudly, overheard by myself and the man repairing the telephone, I got more and more angry with his lack of contact with her suffering.

In the room nearest to where I sat, reserved for those patients needing most nursing care, was a man, Walter. Although I had never seen him, I had been aware of him in the earlier sessions because of the fact that he called the nurses frequently for help. When they went into his room, they seemed to have difficulty in understanding what he wanted, partly because of his deafness and partly because of his confusion. Over the previous two weeks, access to his room had become limited by a barrier-nursing policy which necessitated staff wearing rubber gloves and a face mask when entering his room. In the previous sessions he had not rung his call bell once.

*This day I thought a lot about Walter during the observation. Again there was silence from his room. I was filled with a longing to go in and touch him. A nurse switched on the light in his room. The light switches were on the wall outside the rooms. I waited for someone to go in and be with him. I delayed my departure to see if someone would go in. No one did. His isolation was unbearable.*

## Shuttering off

In the weeks following Walter's death I found myself shuttering-off from the realities around me, much as the ward had been shuttered off for the removal of a body.

I had strongly to resist the urge to do something, to be busy or useful. It was particularly difficult when people were calling out for help and no one came immediately, to tolerate my role as an observer.

*Once, a woman in the room nearest to me called out. It was a few minutes before the nurse came, to discover that she had fallen out of bed. I felt guilty and resented the role that kept me from responding.*

I occupied myself by labelling people and assigning them roles as staff, patients, visitors, volunteers, in an attempt to make meaning out of the situation. I was comforted by familiar faces doing familiar routines, such as the regular appearance of the 'foot'-woman, who did her rounds with a basket and stool offering chiropody and manicures. When a label would not fit comfortably, I was disconcerted.

*In one observation, I was shocked by a very young, very thin girl coming out of a room. My initial label was 'patient', but my mind rebelled and refused to think about this possibility and instantly reassigned her as a relative.*

I became excited by the development of a philosophy about the place. The unit was named after a butterfly and the staff wore butterfly badges and logos. It had been explained to me that their philosophy was that although a patient's life in the unit may be brief it could be bright like that of a butterfly. Based on my observations I revised this. The rooms were cocoons, the patients were caterpillars, their bodies slowly disintegrating to undergo a transformation at death, into butterflies, the symbol of the spirit. This theory had me moving onto thoughts about the ideal environment for a caterpillar and how to supply it. Through these ruminations, I was protected from recognition of what was actually happening to the people in the unit.

I was reluctant to get emotionally involved again.

*Another man was in Walter's room, and in the other room close to me, Salee, an Indian woman with a shaven head, who was unable to communicate verbally with the nurses, sat bolt upright in her bed, her back to the door. I did not want to think about what might be in her mind. I thought about the role of the cat in the unit for a whole hour. I felt sleepy and disassociated, lulled by the sound of the air conditioning.*

When it came to writing up a final account of the observations I initially produced a scientific medical paper. On rewriting it, I found it emotionally difficult to give a detailed account of what I had seen and felt. It was not until I had done this that I came close to recognising the extent of my fear of helplessness.

## In touch again

It was seeing warm human contact again that restored me. This also put me back in touch with the painful reality of dying.

### Session 10

*An Afro-Caribbean woman said goodbye to a visitor at the door of one of the rooms. She stood in her slippers, as she would at her own front door. After the visitor had left, she walked over to two of the nurses at the nurses' station and hugged each of them around the waist and, still with her arm around one of them, they talked. There was a smiling acceptance of the difficulties she faced as her husband lay dying, shared warmly between them.*

*A tall, thin, elderly man making his way back from a telephone call paused at the door of another elderly man who came out to speak with him. They exchanged a few details about their stay in the unit. Their isolation and physical frailty acknowledged, they tentatively arranged to visit each other's rooms later. The polite exchange held the companionship of meeting a fellow sufferer.*

*A young overweight Indian woman was accompanied into the corridor by her husband. He went to unfold the wheelchair outside her room. She shook her head and continued, walking painfully slowly with the aid of a walking frame. The frame marked the carpet as she dragged it along. The back of her night-dress was blood-stained. I felt angry. If they had to be in hospital, this couple belonged in a maternity unit, not here.*

*As I left, I had a glimpse of Salee, shaven headed, at the edge of her bed silently struggling to get out. Her bare legs tangled in the raised cot sides of the bed.*

*There was a wooden walking stick stuck into a bin outside the back door. Well worn, it had a slight crack. I took it with me wondering why it had been discarded and what had happened to the person who had owned it.*

## Conclusion: holding the balance

During the weeks of the observation, I underwent a process. Initial anxiety, coupled with loneliness and isolation, as I found myself without the protection of my professional role and defences. The nightmare of helplessness in the face of the reality of death, followed by the pain of dying in isolation.

Then I built the defences to protect myself again and shut off emotional contact. Only towards the end could I allow myself to get in touch again both with the pain and the human warmth of support.

This personal experience within one particular unit will not apply universally. Much of what I felt was my own personal reaction to being there.

The overwhelming nature of the experience required a period of reflection to digest what I had been confronted with. I wondered, if this was the impact of being an observer on the unit for one hour a week what must it be like for those who worked there for many hours a day without any opportunity to reflect on what was happening to them. Some of what I had found myself doing, the urge to act, to label, to philosophise, in order to protect myself was reflected in the unit. The urgency to do something, to be of some use, was reflected in the business of the staff who rarely sat still, pacing the corridor vigilantly. They attempted to label me in various ways, usually anxiously enquiring as to whether I was waiting for someone.

One nurse who knew that I was there as an observer expressed how disconcerting my presence was. The presence of someone who was attempting to see what happened went against a culture where emotions were shuttered off. The unit had a philosophy of care which, while not of a specifically religious nature as in many hospices, was proposed as a model and was supported by butterfly badges and emblems. A tendency to cut off emotional reality was most marked in the manner in which the body was removed from the ward. It was also reflected in the lack of use of the day room as a communal room and in the emphasis on the privacy of the patients' rooms. These opportunities, offered by the culture of the unit for personal defensiveness, allowed the individual a retreat from the experience of being there and formed part of a social defence system.

Both staff and patients in such a unit are faced with the dilemma of maintaining warm human contact that truly expresses the reality of facing death, while at the same time keeping sufficient distance to prevent being overwhelmed by it. There needs to be an acknowledgement of the need for support, while maintaining a respect for privacy. This balance needs to be held by the patient according to his or her changing needs over time. The temptation is for it to be held by the staff, in some instances erring on the side of too much privacy, leaving the patient alone and isolated. In general, in a hospice the major issues of death and dying facing the patient and their family are very much on the agenda and are dealt with in a much more open way than in most hospital settings. However, the situation may be acknowledged and openly discussed, but the emotion connected with it remains 'shuttered off' or split off. The staff may find that in order to protect themselves from the distress of their close work with the dying they need to cut themselves off from the painful affects created by the situation. This may in turn leave them unable to make contact with patients who are struggling with the same difficulty.

Within the unit, these defences may have become part of the culture, making it difficult for staff or patients to exist outside of them. My own emotional development from being overwhelmed, to defensiveness, to being able to be more in touch again, may reflect a continual oscillation in the culture of the unit between procedural support, retreat into isolationist privacy and the emergence of a more sensitive contact. In a wider context, this particular unit may suffer from its close proximity to a district general hospital which may want to maintain the hospice as an isolation unit, thus splitting itself off from its dying patients. Moves towards more community based care and the integration of palliative care teams within the hospital setting may help to overcome some of these tendencies, but working with the dying will always stir up painful emotions and anxiety. Until professionals acknowledge the impact on themselves of working closely with dying patients, they are unlikely to recognise its impact on their clinical practice.

## References

Hinshelwood RD and Skogstad W (2000). The method of observing organisations. In: Hinshelwood RD and Skogstad W, ed. *Observing Organisations: Anxiety, Defence and Culture in Health Care*. Routledge, London, pp. 17–26.

Menzies I ([1958] 1988). The functioning of social systems as a defence against anxiety. A report on a study of the nursing service of a general hospital. In: Menzies Lyth I.

*Containing Anxiety in Institutions. Selected Essays Volume I.* Free Association Books, London, pp. 463–475.

Ramsay N (2000). Sitting close to death: a palliative care unit. In: Hinshelwood RD and Skogstad W, ed. *Observing Organisations: Anxiety, Defence and Culture in Health Care.* Routledge, London, pp. 142–152.

Saunders CM (1960). *Care of the Dying.* Macmillan, London.

Speck P (1970). Visiting in a female psycho-geriatric ward. *British Journal of Psychiatry* **117**, 93–94.

# 7

# Maintaining a healthy team

*Peter Speck*

## Introduction: concerning conscious and unconscious processes

Janet was a ward sister in a general hospital and had been a senior nurse for >25 years. She was a respected member of staff and known to be quite strict in the way in which she guided and trained her junior staff. Her ward was part of a very busy surgical unit where patients went to theatre for a variety of complex operations. Many of these patients returned to her ward following radical surgery or 'open and close' procedures for inoperable tumours. Some patients would soon become terminally ill and the ward sister would assign a colleague to provide 'special' care until such time as that person died. If the assigned nurse became distressed, then Janet would inform her of the need to 'toughen up' and not become so emotionally involved. One day, a patient returned from theatre and, as no-one else was available, it fell to Janet to do the observations. As she was standing by the patient, he developed a severe haemorrhage and vomited blood all over her, before dying. Janet ran to the sluice room and was found by the staff nurse to be shaking violently and sobbing uncontrollably. It later emerged that when Janet was a junior nurse, she had experienced a similarly traumatic death of a patient whom she had got to know very well. The patient had been very like her own brother who had emigrated some years before and who she very much missed. When that patient died, she had been extremely distressed. Her ward sister at the time had told Janet the patient meant nothing to her and that she was over-reacting and proceeded to tell her off, in the middle of a large open 'Nightingale' ward, for being an emotional wreck and a disgrace. Janet 'buried' her distress and vowed never to put herself in that position again. When she subsequently became a ward sister, she made sure always to assign another nurse to care for any patient likely to die suddenly so that Janet could defend herself by avoiding the situation. On this particular day, the post-operative patient who haemorrhaged over her reactivated the memory of 30 years before and compounded the distress she would already have felt for this sudden and upsetting death.

Janet illustrates very clearly how events in the present, in the 'here and now', can sometimes give rise to a reaction which is over and above what one would expect when reviewing the situation objectively. The reaction has been reinforced by the painful suppressed memory that she had defended herself from revisiting.

During the course of our normal human growth and development, we have a variety of experiences which help to shape our behaviour and our personality in later life. Some of those experiences may be emotionally or psychologically painful and lead us to bury them deep in our unconscious mind in the hope that, even if they do not go away, we can at least forget them.

These aspects of ourselves influence our conscious processes in terms of our relationships with individuals and our behaviour in groups. We operate at two levels—the conscious and the unconscious—and often we give a symbolic meaning to the unconscious mental life. For this reason, a comment at a conscious level may also, at the unconscious level, have a symbolic significance for the individual. For example, a complaint about the distribution of car parking space has a clear valid meaning at a conscious level, but may also be seen unconsciously as a symbolic communication concerning a management that gives little value to other staff members and their needs. Similarly, a group of staff who discuss the problems they experience with the switchboard may also be referring, unconsciously, to a breakdown in communication between departments or between team members. The emotions generated in both these examples can lead to a great sense of frustration and powerlessness which may not be attended to at the level required within the team or the organization.

A team or organization, like the individuals within it, will develop defences against any emotions which may be perceived as too difficult or too painful to acknowledge, and may have a variety of ways of avoiding any real engagement.

## Influences on emotional response

*Events outside of the organization* may generate considerable emotion as a result of, for example, new government policy, changes to local health structures or in society's attitudes towards hospitals or medical staff.

An example of this was the difficulty experienced by UK pathologists who felt themselves to be under attack by families and society following the scandal at Alder-Hey Children's Hospital in Liverpool, concerning the retention of organs from deceased persons following autopsy (Redfern 2001). In some cases, the attack was real, but for many the reaction was to a perceived threat resulting from media coverage and the possibility that pathologists would be required to conduct face to face interviews with distressed families, for which they felt ill-trained. Some also felt they were 'bad people' because of the nature of their work and comments made by friends and others. Following Alder-Hey, it became clear that the attitudes of many people in society had moved from 'not wanting to know' to actually wanting far more detail regarding a post-mortem examination, so that they could make informed decisions about the autopsy and their wishes in connection with tissues and organs removed for examination. Moving from an overprotective, paternalistic, approach when dealing with distressed relatives to a more consultative form of discussion required staff to value the emotions expressed by families and develop the skills to respond to them more appropriately. It also meant that staff began to reflect on and acknowledge the effects of the work on themselves and the distress they sometimes had to contain for themselves and others.

*Sources of conflict within the organization* may create powerful feelings and lead people to defend against them. Examples of sources of conflict include those sometimes generated by a 'perceived distant' management and their staff who have direct patient contact; or between groups and departments in competition for resources—such as office space or the training budget. Defences against emotion can be healthy and provide an important means of managing stress and anxiety, as part of personal and professional growth. However, some defences which operate at a team or organizational level can block any contact with reality and actively take staff away from the primary task they are there to address, and often prevent their engaging with any change agenda as they move defensively into 'survival' mode. If one looks at descriptions of some caring organizations, the first view can be of a variety of organizational charts, flow charts and mission statements. These may be much more about processes than about people, and the descriptors and titles used may be very functional and devoid of anything that might smack of emotion, in case it gives the impression of a 'touchy-feely' enterprise.

Denial is the most obvious defence as it requires the individual or organization to push away or 'bury' certain experiences, thoughts and feelings from conscious awareness because they create too much anxiety as described in Box 7.1.

The fact that many in-patient hospices and specialist palliative care units are a business is unpalatable to some, but represents a reality if adequate resources are to be secured in order that quality personalized care can be delivered to patients and families. The tension between the business ethos and the caring image can be painful for staff who have entered this aspect of health care as an expression of their personal beliefs or life philosophy. In particular, the tension may be resolved by colluding with what I have termed the 'chronic niceness'

---

**Box 7.1** DENIAL AS A DEFENCE AGAINST ANXIETY OF CHANGE

---

An example would be of an organization which fails to recognize the possible change in funding stream which could result from the opening of a new service provider (e.g. Hospice 'A') in a neighbouring health area, geographically close to the edge of the boundary. Commissioners and patients may feel that the new Hospice A is much nearer to some populations which currently look to Hospice B for care and may consider commissioning palliative care services with Hospice A and switching from Hospice B. Failure to recognize this possibility and address the issue could lead to a funding crisis for Hospice B which would then have a great impact on staff and the service they provide. If the organization fails to address this reality on the assumption that they are a tried and tested service who have always been supported by the Primary Care Trust and the community, and so do not need to do anything, they could be in for a shock. A dialogue needs to be opened between Hospice A and Hospice B to look at how the needs of the patients within their respective geographical areas may best be met and the extent to which a collaborative approach would help where their two boundaries meet. The person who attempts to suggest such an approach either may meet considerable resistance and feel unheard, or they may be sent off to explore the feasibility of collaboration. The reality of uncertainty about the future and probable necessity for change may eventually break through the earlier complacency and denial and could force the organization (Hospice B) to deal with some even more powerful emotions than those they denied in the beginning as they look to rationalize services and contemplate staff redundancies.

fantasy. By this is meant the way in which the individual and aspects of the organization collude to split off and deny negative aspects of caring daily for dying people and the fact that this is undertaken in what is also a business context. The fantasy that is created is that 'the staff are nice people, who are caring for really nice dying people, who are going to have a nice death in a nice place. This protects everyone from facing the fact that the relationship between the carers and the dying can often arouse very primitive and powerful feelings which are disturbingly "not-nice" ' (Speck 1984, p. 97). This fantasy enables staff to maintain a sense of cohesiveness and solidarity which allows them to deny any negative feelings about their patients or each other! Many of the negative feelings that are split-off get projected outside of the team or the hospice onto the management group, or the hospice council, or their sponsoring charity/NHS purchasers who 'don't seem to understand what we are about and only look at results and the financial bottom line'. Projecting negative feelings onto others, such as the family, can help us to feel more comfortable in seeing the patient–staff relationship as positive and, where there are difficulties, to imagine these could be resolved if the family were only 'more caring'. The criticisms of care voiced by a family may not then be heard or may be dismissed as vindictive or punitive and 'only to be expected from that sort of family'.

The above, however, may be clearly rooted in reality in that perhaps senior management really does not seem to value the staff, or the expectations of the charity or government are unrealistic without additional resources, and Mr Jones' family really are 'the family from hell'. Unless there is a mechanism in place regularly to appraise the emotional effects upon staff of the work they do, and the organizational dynamic, the staff's morale and self-image of themselves as caring, competent and nice people will be hard to sustain. As a result, they can lose touch with what is reality and what is fantasy. Building and sustaining the team(s) who provide palliative care should be a regular aspect of the team's life, as described in Chapter 8, and not something which only takes place in the face of team or organizational crises.

## Importance of the social group

A dynamic is created at team, departmental and organizational level which will affect the way in which individuals perform at work. There will also be an inter-relationship with how the individual behaves in their social life and at home. It is important not to ignore the effectiveness of the social or 'sentient' groupings for reinforcing, or undermining, the life of the team in a variety of ways. Much strengthening of team relationships can occur away from the workplace where people can offer to support each other in an informal way and develop confidence and trust in each other as people. Conversely, within a social setting, one can discover how irritating or boring someone can be away from their work role. For those in management positions, it is important to manage the transition from work role to social role and to recognize that the boss is still the boss even in a relaxed setting. Confusion about this can create misunderstanding and feelings of betrayal if, at work, the manager has to discipline a staff member who had come to perceive them as a friend and not a manager. One of the difficult aspects of leadership is the way in which one is in the team yet not fully of the team because of the need to maintain a degree of distance to free oneself to function as a manager when required. The social or sentient grouping can also be a place where the negatives are given expression in a way they may not be at work meetings. People who may be silent in the work meeting may be quite vocal in the canteen or the pub and decisions previously agreed can effectively be overturned outside the team meeting. This is important for leadership as it relates directly to issues of power and authority (see Chapter 5 of this volume).

Not all emotional reactions in the 'here and now' experience are related to earlier stages of our development or to painful past experiences. Sometimes we react emotionally because we recognize the signs in a relationship or encounter that the conversation is moving in a familiar direction based on direct experience of the people concerned. Thus the phone ringing at half past four on a Friday afternoon may be a doctor or nurse ringing the palliative care team to refer a patient before that doctor or nurse goes off for the weekend. The fact that this may be a regular occurrence on a Friday afternoon from that particular ward may generate a degree of emotional response in the palliative care team member who picks up the phone. We can interpret the different possible emotional responses in various ways.

From a psychoanalytical perspective, we may suggest that some of the reaction could be related to experiences of a parent who would suddenly express of the child an expectation that they were previously not aware of and now must accommodate. However, the reaction is just as likely to be generated because it is another example of lack of forethought by the ward staff when making a late referral that should have been made earlier in the day following the morning ward round.

From a cognitive viewpoint, we might say that as reason develops, we become more aware of emotion as we try to make sense of what we are seeing or hearing. There needs to be some form of appraisal of the experience and it is in the act of appraising that we generate, and become aware of, an emotional response. In this example, the palliative care team member is drawing on their experience of the ward team, their memory of previous Friday afternoon referrals and the effect of late referrals which require him/her to reschedule the end of day's work, recognizing that this could have been obviated by an earlier phone call. Anxiety and frustration may arise and either be contained, diverted onto someone else in the office by *displacement*, or be given expression by 'exploding' at the ward staff member making the phone call. How the interaction is handled will depend on the way in which the event is 'appraised'. Lazarus (2001) describes two levels of appraisal: primary and secondary.

- At the primary level, the palliative care team member is thinking 'Does this affect me personally, or am I in trouble or likely to benefit from this in the future?'
- At the secondary level, the person thinks 'What can I do about it, and how can I cope?'

Depending on the appraisal, the individual may decide that containing their own feelings, accepting the referral and going to review the patient on the ward before going home might put them in good standing with their palliative care colleague who is 'on call' Friday evening. This might also help team processes and relationships. Alternatively, he/she could simply log the referral and leave it on the desk for their colleague before going home, or perhaps go up to the ward and complain to the staff about late referrals and their effect on others. Thinking it through (as part of the process of appraisal) will often affect the emotion that is felt and how, if at all, it is expressed.

The person's social context will play a part because it is within a social milieu that we learn emotional norms and forms of expression. Various settings will provide us with the necessary language, scripts and roles by which we can express our emotional responses to a variety of experiences. For some people, this social milieu will be rich, but for others it is very impoverished and they may struggle both to understand and to know how to express what they are feeling. The organization itself will also have developed a culture within which certain norms of behaviour have been created. These norms will also relate to what emotions may be expressed, and how, within the various aspects of organizational life. It follows that there will be norms of behaviour within teams together with ways of managing emotion, ranging from denial to full and free expression. Thus, in the example given, the response to the ward staff may be tempered by the team's cultural norms of how they do or do not manage conflict, and the importance they attach to always being thought of as 'nice'.

## The effects of the work

Unless you work as a funeral director, a palliative care specialist, in the emergency services or in certain branches of health care, death will not feature very frequently in your life experience. It is for this reason that the people who become caught up in a major incident, where a large number of people die or are seriously injured, may be severely traumatized by their overexposure to death. The DSM-IVTR (2002) recognizes such trauma as requiring specialist intervention to address the issues of acute anxiety created by such events.

Grief experienced as a result of a personal bereavement is closely related to the nature of the relationship with the deceased and the role the deceased had in the life of the survivor. We recognize that this is a natural response, and with appropriate help and support the bereaved individual is able, in time, to incorporate the deceased into their ongoing life and develop a new identity for themselves. For most, this encounter with death does not happen too often, until one reaches the age where a great deal of time may be spent attending funerals of friends and relatives.

What of the professional carer who in the course of their work frequently attends people who are dying and therefore faces death weekly if not daily? How do they cope with this abnormal exposure to mortality and still function within their professional role? (Chapter 6 provides an interesting and important observation study of some of the effects of working in a hospice environment).

This is not solely an issue for palliative care staff, as Vachon has indicated (1995). However, working closely with dying people can put one in touch with previous loss experience and reawaken unresolved grief which may affect how one relates to the person being cared for in the present. Some of the unresolved grief reactions may be in relation to past patients who have been cared for, and who have left an impression on the carer which created a sense of loss at the time of their death but may not have been acknowledged or addressed then or later (see Box 7.2).

If our role at work involves caring for people who are going to die, it is likely that some of these people will have an effect upon us. Not every patient will do this since we do not form significant *affectional bonds* (positive or negative) with everyone (Bowlby 1969). However, we cannot predict which people will engender powerful feelings within us. Sometimes it is a clear attraction between two people who respond warmly to each other, in other cases it may be that the patient reminds us of a family member or significant person in our life for whom we have strong feelings of dislike, liking or ambivalence. Colleagues may not recognize that this has happened and may place a greatly reduced value on the relationship, which may not permit any expression of feeling following the patient's death, as in the case of the ward sister Janet. This can be compounded if the cultural norm of the team or organization is one of non-expression of feeling at any time.

---

**Box 7.2** UNRESOLVED OR DELAYED GRIEF

---

Carol was a 24-year-old nurse who worked on an oncology ward caring for patients with leukaemia. Many of the patients were of a similar age to Carol and she established a good rapport with them, was popular and seen as a very capable and reliable member of staff. Some of 'her' patients responded well to treatment and went into remission, but sometimes the disease would return and they would be readmitted for further, often aggressive, treatment. Carol was able to offer effective support to these patients on the first few admissions, but found it much harder when the disease returned and hope was diminishing of any future remission. During one particular month, there had been a large number of deaths on the ward, some of them quite distressing to Carol as she felt ambivalent about continuing aggressive therapy when she believed the person was close to death. Because the ward was very busy with lots of new admissions and shortage of staff, there was little opportunity for Carol to attend to her own emotional needs. Carol believed that if you offered good care it should enable people to have a 'good death' and yet this had not been the case for several of 'her' patients.

One evening she went to a club with some friends and drank quite heavily. During a lull in the music, Carol staggered into the centre of the dance floor and began to shout at people 'How can you enjoy yourselves like this. Don't you know there's young people of our age dying at this moment. Don't you care? ... etc.' Then she fell down on the floor and sobbed. Her friends looked after her and took her home. Subsequently, talking to a counsellor, Carol recognized that she was not having a 'nervous breakdown'. She had found herself unable any more to 'contain' the unresolved grief she had been carrying for a long list of patients she had cared for and who had died in ways she had not wished for them. She had overidentified with some of her patients and lost her capacity to cope because of the emotional overload. Her perception of herself as a competent, caring, person had shattered and she now felt that she was a 'bad' person who 'killed off' the people she liked and cared for. While this was a fantasy and *not* the reality, it was very real to Carol at the time. Later she recognized the importance of attending to feelings aroused by the work on a regular basis and was instrumental in setting up a multiprofessional staff support group on her unit.

---

If the professional carer does not know and understand the nature of their own responses to other people, they can easily find themselves responding to the patient *as if* they were that family member or personal friend. This is part of an unconscious process termed *transference* by which we respond to another person as if they were the other person we wish them to be. If the other then responds by accepting the transference and 'becomes for us' that other person, the relationship has moved from a purely professional one into something closer to an intimate personal relationship through what is termed the *counter-transference* (Cairns 1996). Transference is not something occurring exclusively in a counselling/therapeutic relationship but is experienced in many of our interpersonal encounters and can influence how we behave towards other people in a variety of settings. In the context of palliative care, however, it can be important to develop the skill of recognizing when it is happening in order to maintain ourselves in the professional role. This is but one example of how an unconscious process can influence behaviour by 'sucking' us out of role, with consequent loss of boundary management.

'Splitting' is another common way of managing the tensions sometimes created by working with people with life-threatening disease. In the case of Carol, she worked in a unit where the medical team were very focused on aggressive treatment modes which achieved success for some but not for all. They always hoped for cure or a potential 'breakthrough' in conquering the disease. To some extent, they were distanced from the patient as a person and saw the patient who died as a 'failure'. One transplant surgeon commented to me, a few days after performing a transplant, 'That liver is doing fantastically well—it's a shame the guy has just died'. It is not that the medical team do not care about the person, but the human caring aspect is split off and vested in the nurse, chaplain or others who remain close to the patient and become identified with all that is good, loving and nice. Therefore, when the patient dies, the nurse or other colleague who was close to the patient can become the recipient of the doctor's anger and frustration at the perceived failure. This can be enhanced by an unconscious rivalry between doctor and nurse linked to 'a covert competitiveness for the gratitude of the patient, who may seem to have shrugged off dependency and asserted his or her autonomy in the only way left—by dying' (Speck, 1984, p. 96). For Carol, who could no longer hold on to a self-image as being good, loving and nice, any implied or expressed criticism from the medical team about the care of *their* patient who had died would have been hard to deal with. Within palliative care, there is an attempt to hold this split (and the ambivalence of being both a 'good' and a 'bad' object) by working towards a partnership between doctor, nurse, other team members and patient within an interdisciplinary team. However, strong feelings may still be around and influence the way in which team members address their primary task of caring for patients and working effectively with each other in delivering that care.

## Joining and leaving a team

If a multi- or interdisciplinary team has been working together for some time, they will have developed ways of working together, an element of trust in each other and knowledge of each other's strengths and weaknesses. They will also have established a way of doing things and have assigned (and assumed) roles within the team which can make it difficult for a new person to join. A degree of robustness can be a useful asset in applicants seeking to work in an interdisciplinary team.

In staff selection, the resourcefulness of applicants needs to be assessed as well as their professional competence and expertise. Is the candidate sufficiently mature and secure in their own professional identity to free them to work in a flexible way within a team? If not, the person may feel very isolated (especially if they are the only representative of that professional group within the team) and could become territorially defensive. A non-team player can become quite a disruptive force within the team but, in reality, not all professionals learn team skills as they move through their career, and much learning may need to take place within the team. Respect for others, and the ability to trust and support colleagues is important—together with a sense of humour which will often save a team from disintegrating through internal conflict. Dynamically, although probably interviewed and appointed in collaboration with some team members, the team still need to open up a space for the new person to enter. There can be many different expectations of the new person, and each team member will be watchful of how they do the work and will be assessing their skills and competence. Because the various members of the team will have developed roles and modes of behaving in team meetings, the new person can feel marginalized unless a conscious effort is made to include them. At an unconscious level, the new person symbolizes the one who has gone and for whom there may be a sense of loss or relief. Staff who join an existing team require time to learn not just the ways of working, but also the way in which the various interactions will affect how they feel or react, or pretend to feel, in order to maintain the team cohesiveness or be 'accepted' by others. Just as we 'take up our role at work', so we also take up an emotional script that may become attached to that role. Taking up a role which gives little freedom to show personal emotional responses openly (as for example the role of a bereavement officer) does not mean that feelings are not being generated and experienced within the person. The constraints of the role may, depending on the strengths and weaknesses of the role bearer, lead to emotion being displaced onto others at other times in an inappropriate way.

It is similar when people leave a team. If they have been part of the team for a long time, they will have acquired an emotional as well as a work role within the team. In some teams, the forces holding people together are such that to contemplate leaving can feel like a betrayal. To choose to apply for another job can be perceived as a rejection. One team member commented 'I think the only way I could legitimately leave this team is by dying'. Other team members have great ambivalence about somebody leaving unless it is because of ill health, marriage or death. Promotion may generate a mixture of congratulations, pleasure in another's success, jealousy or envy. If this happens at a time of budgetary pressures and a recruitment freeze, the negatives may surface as the implications of the loss become clear, thus ensuring that the leaver feels guilty for precipitating the crisis. Ambivalence can also be around when a colleague retires, especially if the person is taking early retirement as this can also be experienced as a rejection. Many of these feelings may remain unspoken but may need to be acknowledged if the separation is to happen in a non-punitive fashion.

It can be helpful, if it is not already happening on a regular basis, for someone to help the team address their own dynamic issues as a regular part of working together. As Payne in Chapter 8 of this volume indicates, this is much easier if it happens as part and parcel of the team's ongoing life and work.

## Managing stress and conflict

### The importance of clinical supervision

The importance of supervising clinical practice has been recognized in the field of psychotherapy and other psychological therapies since the 1920s (Doehrman 1976), though other areas of clinical practice were slower to establish supervision as an essential component of care. Seventy years later, in *'A Vision for the Future'* (1993), the UK Department of Health advocated that the concept and appropriateness of clinical supervision should be explored further and a report made to the professions.

Clinical supervision was seen as 'a formal process of professional support and learning which enables individual practitioners to develop knowledge and competence, assume responsibility for their own practice and enhance consumer protection and safety of care in complex clinical situations' (Department of Health 1993). In the ensuing years, various models of supervision, mentorship and interpersonal support were developed. Research studies began to show the efficacy of clinical supervision (e.g. Butterworth *et al.* 1996) though the paucity of good empirical evidence was also highlighted (Yegdich and Cushing 1998). The arrival of clinical governance as 'the means by which organizations ensure the provision of quality clinical care by making individuals accountable for setting, maintaining and monitoring performance standards' (Department of Public Health 1998) effectively placed responsibility for quality of care jointly on organizations and on individuals within those organizations. Participating in clinical supervision demonstrates clearly that the individual is exercising their responsibility under clinical governance, as well as the organization having a clear responsibility to support access by clinical staff to appropriate supervision. Within palliative care, there has been a long tradition of providing staff support activities in various forms and with varied degrees of success. The multidisciplinary nature of palliative care has meant that clinical supervision benefits from being multidisciplinary as many of the issues in clinical practice are multifaceted and benefit from such an approach. Uni-disciplinary meetings may also be required.

While the aims of clinical supervision continue to be debated, Brocklehurst (1994) identifies some common features of the supervision relationship being of fundamental importance. Brocklehurst also highlights the importance of structure and process, and the fact that it needs to be an active process with equal input from supervisor and supervisee. Related aims include ensuring safe practice, developing skills, encouraging personal and professional growth and supporting staff. The word 'support' is significant because it raises one of the sources of confusion when thinking about ways of managing stress within and between teams. Supervision is primarily concerned with the professional development of the supervisee(s) and the relationship of care with and for patients (Yegdich 1999). Any therapeutic benefit for individual team members is secondary to the main aim of clinical supervision. Similarly, there can be confusion, and suspicion, around 'staff support groups' which may be perceived as having a personal therapeutic role. However, the focus of such groups should have a clearly agreed and understood task of being work related and not an opportunity for 'sorting each other out' or intruding into the private life of individual members. This does not mean that such 'support' meetings or clinical supervision meetings cannot be experienced as supportive, because this is one aspect of their purpose. If such groups are to be able to reduce rather than enhance stress in the workplace and work relationships, there needs to be clarity of task and well-managed boundaries which are held by the facilitator/ supervisor.

## *Other opportunities to address stress and conflict*

There are various ways in which stress and conflict may be addressed. Many of the stressful events which occur in the life of the team may be addressed in the context of clinical supervision, or within a specific staff support group, or as a natural part of any other team meeting where opportunity is provided for 'debriefing' or addressing any issues relating to team dynamics. A key factor is making the time and space to meet together, or allocating time on occasions when already meeting.

If the team is located together on one site, it is clearly easier for them to meet more regularly. In respect of palliative care provision in the community, it is equally, if not more, important for the community staff who offer the service to meet together to develop and maintain a team identity. If their geographical area is large and that makes it difficult to meet physically together with any frequency, it is important to explore other ways of maintaining contact and communication. This might include the use of E-mail, telephone and video/ telephone conference calls as well as ensuring that when they do meet (for a training or business meeting), some time is allocated for social activity and attention to working relationships. Depending on the size of the team, the configuration of meetings will also vary as it will not be appropriate, or feasible, for everyone to attend every meeting. Many meetings will be business focused and may be concerned with managerial issues: the strategic plan, the business plan, health and safety, fire lectures, developing and reviewing policies, etc. Other meetings will be of a more clinical nature: the ward round, case reviews, journal club, clinical supervision and updates. Within some of these meetings, there may be opportunity to reflect on the dynamic of the meeting, but in reality this is not very likely and people may come out of meetings with a variety of different feelings that they may or may not feel able to express—except in the canteen or car park later. Whether the team is based in a hospital, a hospice or in the wider community outside, it can be beneficial to allocate some time each week or month when the team specifically focus on their own interactions, and share and discuss how they feel in respect of the life of the team and the work they are doing. This may be at a specially convened meeting or an allocated slot as part of the agenda for another meeting. This is not a waste of time or self-indulgent navel-gazing, but an essential component for maintaining a healthy team life. Sometimes the team can undertake this task for themselves, but there will also be times when they will need to use an outside facilitator. Clearly there are many different ways of achieving this type of discussion, and a degree of trust and safety is required if people are to be able to be honest and constructive in what they share. Clarifying the task for the meeting (or for that section of the meeting if part of another meeting) is crucial so that there is no confusion about the agenda being 'work focused' and not an opportunity for personal therapy or personal attacks.

The primary focus should be work-related issues. If, in the process, it emerges that there is a personal problem or crisis for a team member, which is affecting how they are at work, then that person needs to acknowledge it and seek appropriate help and support elsewhere. It is not, I believe, the task of the team to move into 'sorting out X or Y's personal life'. This does not mean that the team cannot be generally supportive of the personal stress and problems of a colleague. The team meeting may need to discuss ways of easing X's workload for a period or accepting a period of variable work hours until the crisis is over. The main task of any support/team review meeting should remain clear: to reflect on the effect of the work on the person's role and any

**Table 7.1** Factors tending to create conflict (after Cummings 1998)

1. Ambiguous role boundaries, roles that are changing, protective territorialism
2. Interdisciplinary professional rivalry
3. Communication barriers
4. Leadership style not congruent with needs of team
5. Decision making that excludes some team members
6. Team members with different goals, expectations
7. Displaced hostility, previous conflicts
8. Differing personality styles
9. Continuing change threatening roles or affecting team members unequally
10. Scarcity of resources.

influences on their relationships with other team members. There needs to develop an understanding that people can discuss freely and without judgement. However, this is an ideal not always realized without a measure of competent external facilitation.

Cummings (1998) provides a clear picture of the ways in which conflict can arise within the interdisciplinary team. She outlines the factors that may lead to conflict (Table 7.1) and the variables which may affect the way the conflict may manifest and develop (Table 7.2).

Cummings suggests that understanding these factors can enhance the chance of a healthy resolution rather than destructive confrontation, and she states the important truth that conflict cannot be resolved until it is acknowledged. Again this is a challenge for those in a leadership position for it is important that they engage with these issues, decide on the importance of the conflict, and make a decision on whether to ignore them or address them if the team is to remain focused on what they are there to do (see Chapter 5 of this volume).

Often conflict is a manifestation of stress within the team, or within the organization that is then being experienced within the team. Just as the team develops a dynamic and experiences unconscious processes, so does the organization as a whole. Issues at the level of 'top management' or board level may well filter down through the organization and influence the functioning of teams and groups at various points. Often this can be traced to issues of

**Table 7.2** Variables affecting how conflict may develop (after Cummings 1998)

1. Characteristics of individuals involved: motivation, values, aspirations
2. Prior relationship of individuals to each other; a history of difficulty will predict poorer outcome than a history of trust
3. Nature of the problem and value invested in the issue leading to conflict
4. Social environment; is the team fatigued and stressed or is one person likely to lose face or self-esteem?
5. Is the conflict between two people or a manifestation of a split in the team?
6. Is the conflict focused on issues or has it become personal? Is there any coercion, threats in the communications?
7. What are the gains and losses, precedents set, influences on relationships as a consequence of the conflict?

'ownership' in that various groups may unconsciously choose not to take ownership of particular problems so that decisions are left unmade, thus creating uncertainty, confusion and frustration in others parts of the structure (see Box 7.3).

There is often a tension between who should take responsibility for the management of stress within our working life. Should it be the organization or should it be the individual? There is a degree of interplay between the stress of an employee's private life spilling over into work and affecting how they are at work, but also work tensions which can affect their personal life. In her work on the place of stress in the life of palliative care workers, Mary Vachon (1995) has highlighted, in an important review article, that stress and burnout are by no means universal in palliative care. She attributes this to the fact that from the beginning of the hospice movement there was recognition of the need for good organizational and personal coping strategies to deal with stressors. Stress in the work place seems to derive, in her review, from the work environment, occupational role, patients and families, and illnesses. In respect of the environment, this is either to be accepted as a given, or caregivers need to develop new coping strategies to deal with them (Vachon 2004). Team communication problems feature in numerous studies, and Yancik (1984*a*,*b*) cites

---

**Box 7.3 'OWNERSHIP'**

---

During a regular ward meeting on an oncology ward, it was noted that the ward sister and the medical registrar were 'sniping' at each other throughout the meeting. They usually had a very good working relationship, so this present behaviour was unusual. The trigger seemed to be that the ward sister was accepting new admissions into her ward's empty beds in the evening from other doctors. These patients (from other specialties) were housed overnight until transferred to their proper specialty ward later the next day. However, this meant that patients seen by the registrar in clinic, or booked to come in early morning, did not have a bed on the oncology unit. The ward sister felt under great pressure from the other doctors to house their patients temporarily overnight, and this was supported by the duty manager. She also felt disloyal to her registrar colleague but could see no way out as it was difficult to protect an empty bed in the face of a clear need. The sister and doctor were 'acting out' a dynamic within the organization as a whole because other wards and units were also experiencing similar problems and frustration. The sister had spoken to her nurse manager who said it was the doctor's problem and he should talk to his medical colleague; meanwhile the doctors complained about nursing staff becoming difficult. In reality, the hospital had no bed management policy and no-one with authority and power to address the issue across the organization. While the issue remained 'owned' at ward level, nothing would change and relationships would suffer. The registrar and ward sister decided to seek a meeting with *both* the nurse director and the medical director and to go together. This joint approach was successful in moving ownership to a level in the organization where it could be taken on board and addressed across the organization. A bed manager was recruited and a Trust-wide policy developed. While the future was not totally problem free, a considerable amount of stress and animosity was eased at ward level.

lack of support from one's team colleagues as a key stressor. Vachon (1987) focused on the effect of lack of team stability, intergroup and intragroup conflict and the way in which issues to do with personalities within the team and conflict were more powerful causes of stress than the problems experienced in dealing with patients and families, or death and dying. Communication also features largely in respect of other colleagues in the system—whether they were clinical staff, general practitioners, or managers seeking to implement change or having unrealistic expectations of staff.

### Interteam conflict and relationships

Because palliative care is a specialty, it will, of necessity, often be working alongside a variety of other teams who may have different aims and objectives. The team leader and the members need to develop skills appropriate to interteam working, and Cumming's analysis of factors leading to conflict and the ways in which conflict may manifest itself are equally applicable to interteam relationships. As mentioned above, communication is often a root cause of conflict. The role and purpose may not be clearly understood by the various people involved in providing care. Each may hold assumptions about the other's role, competence and purpose in offering care to a particular patient or family. If that is not explored and clarified, conflict can quickly arise and may be expressed as an interpersonal or interteam problem. The causes can be complex but often centre around competing for resources, poor communication, ambiguity about who is responsible for what, incompatible goals, personality difficulties and previous history. For example, the hospital palliative care team may have been asked to see a patient by the specialist nurse within another team. The consultant may not acknowledge that the time has come to shift the focus from cure to care and may resent any input from palliative care. Both believe they will be acting in the best interests of the patient, but a failure to recognize and address their differences may mean the patient's care becomes a casualty of the conflict.

Sometimes, through meetings between the various parties involved, it is possible to mediate or to reach a compromise. A third party may be needed to facilitate such a meeting. However, this can leave a feeling of dissatisfaction if one party feels they have 'won' or 'lost'. In conflict, people often lose sight of the patient-centred primary task and cannot recognize that each side of the conflict is trying to address the needs of the patient, but from a different perspective. One has only to sit in on a clinical ethics group discussion to recognize that each person is trying to achieve the 'best outcome' for the patient but from very different viewpoints. The development of such groups is an indication of the complexity of some decision making and the difficulty of achieving a consensus without a real dialogue between the various people involved—including the patient and family.

To resolve conflict between teams, or within the wider organization, requires a clear strategy.

- It is important to recognize that there is a conflict and identify the symptoms. Problems and difficulties do not usually go away—even if the one labelled the 'difficult colleague' leaves.
- Recognize the nature and degree of conflict. What is at the heart of the dispute and how serious is it?
- Recognize and understand the sources of conflict. Do some of the people have unrealistic expectations and therefore need to refocus on what is possible? Is the real source of the conflict elsewhere and being 'acted out' within the team?
- Investigate the root cause rather than overfocusing on symptoms.
- Establish the range of possible outcomes.
- Select the desired outcome which removes symptoms and clarify who should be involved in achieving this outcome, e.g. the team leaders of the various teams, senior management, stakeholders, patient representatives, etc.

### Stress is natural, but . . .

Stress management studies indicate that stress is a natural component of human life and can have a motivating aspect, as described by Hans Selye (1956) who used the term 'positive stress' for the sense of being psyched-up as a preliminary to action. Rather than something to be avoided, we actually need it to stimulate effective performance (Orpen 1996). The main cause of damage is when the stress we experience exceeds our capacity to cope over long periods, and thus causes strain. As the stress level increases, we move from a non-engaged state to active engagement with the task and productivity. As stress increases further we reach a point of 'peak performance' beyond which strain begins to manifest itself, panic and desperation ensue and performance falls. From this point, damage also begins to show in terms of physical and psychological breakdown, and is reflected in an increased sickness/absence rate. This progression can be portrayed graphically as an inverted curve, as in Fig. 7.1.

A key factor in much of this is 'control', in that often in the workplace people may feel they have very little control over the volume of work, the pace at which it arrives, or decision-making processes which will affect them and the work they do (Rollinson and Broadfield 2002). When this is coupled with expectations and demands about the quality and quantity of

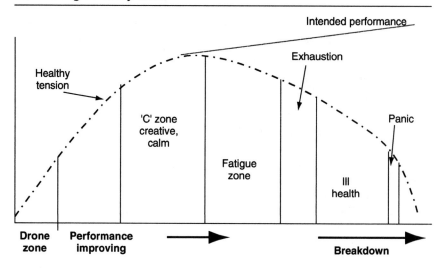

**Fig. 7.1** Zones of the human function curve.

performance, the outcome can range through high achievement, opting out, boredom or exhaustion, as shown in Fig. 7.2.

York (2001) asks whether stress is just a new term to describe work pressure and unhappiness. He believes that stress is more about conflict, confusion and frustration, that the multitasking, balancing of priorities and meeting contradictory demands all generate anxiety which, over time, lead to stress and

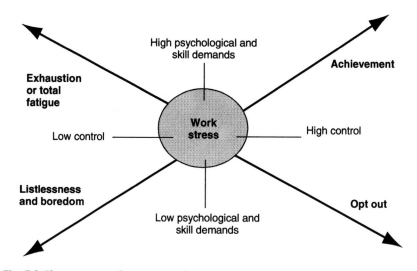

**Fig. 7.2** Elements contributing to work stress.

reduced productivity. Because palliative care tends to attract people with high ideals concerning what they wish to achieve, they can easily fall prey to the desire to be the 'perfect carer'. This can create a great deal of inner stress if the external demands and conditions make it difficult, if not impossible, to maintain the high standard of care they wish to provide, and ultimately this can lead to emotional and psychological exhaustion. I do not like the term 'burnout' because of the connotations of being beyond repair. In many ways, total exhaustion or 'battle fatigue' (Vachon 1988) is a better term because it contains the possibility of rehabilitation and eventual return of the ability to care.

Supporting staff who are experiencing increased levels of stress calls for a multipronged approach. The organization and the team leader need to attend to team building and support (see Chapter 8 of this volume). Staff support groups are of unproven efficacy and their success seems to depend on the quality of facilitation, staff being able to choose the facilitator, the length of time it should run for, and clarifying the task and purpose (Vachon 1987; Finlay 1990). Alexander and Ritchie (1990) show that support from colleagues is also very important, with 67 per cent of the palliative care nurses they interviewed describing how they used 'talking things over with a colleague' as a coping strategy. This compared with 18 per cent who talked with people at home. All this is supported by personal coping strategies which may depend on family support, lifestyle management and the nurturing of a personal philosophy or belief system. The overall picture from the work of Vachon and others is that the incidence of excessive stress is lower than might be expected because of the way in which staff support has always been accepted as an essential component of palliative care. Most stress seems to arise when the coping strategies such as social support, being involved in decision making and work planning, and exercising some control over workload are no longer achievable.

## Conclusion

When one considers the variety of emotional experiences which members of a palliative care team will experience during a working week, it is not surprising to find a variety of expressions of pleasure and frustration within the team when they review the work that they do. Some of the emotional load will be generated outside the team through interaction with patients, families and other professional carers. However, a certain amount will also be generated as a by-product, or toxins, of the dynamic processes that are created within the team itself. Failure to recognize and address the emotional and psychological sequelae of working in palliative care is, I believe, at the heart of much of the staff stress and team difficulties that arise over time. Just as the toxins produced as a result of renal failure require dialysis for their removal, so the dynamic 'toxins' need a form of emotional/psychological 'dialysis' for the well-being of both the individuals and the team as a whole.

A healthy organization is, therefore, one able to acknowledge the presence of an emotional agenda and recognizes that this will operate at both a conscious and an unconscious level. It will also be able to work creatively with the emotion generated by the nature of the work, the internal tensions within the organization and the individual, and thus continue to stay engaged with the main task of the organization, and support the palliative care team in doing the same.

# References

Alexander DA and Ritchie E (1990). 'Stressors' and difficulties in dealing with the terminal patient. *Palliative Medicine* 6(3), 28–33.

Bowlby J (1969). *Attachment and Loss: Attachment*, Vol. I. Basic Books, New York.

Brocklehurst N (1999). An Evaluation Study of Clinical Supervision in Six NHS Trusts. Unpublished PhD Thesis, University of Birmingham.

Butterworth T, Bishop V and Carson J (1996). First steps towards evaluating clinical supervision in nursing and health visiting. Part 1: theory, policy and practice development. *Journal of Clinical Nursing*. 5, 127–132.

Cairns F (1996). Transference and counter-transference. In: Palmer S, Dainow S, Milner P, ed. *Counselling: The BAC Counselling Reader*. Sage, London, pp. 492–499.

Cummings I (1998). The interdisciplinary team. In: Doyle D, Hanks GWC and MacDonald N, ed. *Oxford Textbook of Palliative Medicine*, 2nd edn. Oxford Univeristy Press, Oxford, pp. 19–30.

Department of Health (1993). *A Vision for the Future: Report of the Chief Nursing Officer*. HMSO, London.

Department of Public Health (1998). *Clinical Governance in North Thames: A Paper for Discussion and Consultation*. NHSE North Thames Region Office, London.

Doehrman MJG (1976). Parallel processes in supervision and psychotherapy. *Bulletin of the Manninger Clinic* 40(1), pp. 3–104.

DSM-IVTR (2002). *Diagnostic and Statistical Manual of Mental Disorders*. American Psychiatric Publishing, Arlington, VA.

Finlay IG (1990). Sources of stress in hospice medical directors and matrons. *Palliative Medicine* 4, 5–9.

Lazarus RS and Cohen-Charash Y (2001). Discrete emotions in organisational life. In: Payne RL and Cooper C, ed. *Emotions at Work*. Wiley, Chichester, UK, pp. 45–81.

Orpen C (1996). Want the best? Get stressed! *Chartered Secretary* August, pp. 18–20.

Redfern M (2001). *The Royal Liverpool Children's Inquiry Report*. The Stationery Office, London.

Rollinson D and Broadfield A (2002). *Organizational Behaviour and Analysis*. Pearson Education, Harlow, UK.

Selye H (1956). *The Stress of Life*. McGraw-Hill, New York.

Speck P (1984). Working with dying people. In: Obholzer A, Roberts VZ. *The Unconscious at Work: Individual and Organizational Stress in the Human Services.* Routledge, London.

Vachon MLS (1987). *Occupational Stress in the Care of the Critically Ill, the Dying and the Bereaved.* Hemisphere. New York.

Vachon MLS (1988). Battle fatigue in hospice/palliative care. In: Gilmore A and Gilmore S, ed. *A Safer Death.* Plenum, New York, pp. 149–160.

Vachon MLS (1995). Staff stress in hospice/palliative care: a review. *Palliative Medicine* 9, 91–122.

Vachon MLS (2004). The stress of professional caregivers. In: Doyle D, Hanks G, Cherny NI and Calman K, ed. *Oxford Textbook of Palliative Medicine*, 3rd edn. Oxford University Press, Oxford, pp. 992–1004.

Yancik R (1984a). Sources of work stress for hospice staff. *Journal of Psychosocial Oncology* 2(1), 21–31.

Yancik R (1984b). Coping with hospice work stress. *Journal of Psychosocial Oncology* 2(2), 19–35.

Yegdich T (1999) Lost in the crucible of supportive clinical supervision: supervision is not therapy. *Journal of Advanced Nursing* 29, 1265–1275.

Yegdich T and Cushing A (1998). A historical perspective on clinical supervision in nursing. *Australian and New Zealand Journal of Mental Health Nursing* 7, 3–24.

York P (2001). Getting a grip on stress. *Management Today,* October, p. 105.

# 8

# Team building: how, why and where?

*Malcolm Payne*

## Introduction: everyday team building

The nursing team on one of the wards in the hospice faced difficulties with the mother–son relationship of a female patient dying of liver cancer. The consultant palliative care physician had been called out at night to discuss matters with the son, who had interfered with the syringe driver, because he did not agree with constant medication of his mother. Nurses felt they could no longer cope with the hostile behaviour of the son. People arrived from all over the hospice to make their contribution to the urgent case conference the following morning. The consultant stopped the psychiatrist from getting the history of events from the ward nurse manager. 'Let's wait until everyone's here', he said. 'There are so many complexities involved that it's important we all hear about what's going on.'

This is an example of everyday team building. The consultant made sure that his leadership took into account the communication and planning that everyone in the team would be involved in. He used professional and personal authority and power to emphasize the importance of teamwork, reminding team members of how important it is to strengthen the team's work as part of everything that we do. He took action that enabled the later arrivals to play their part and contribute their voices and knowledge to the decisions made that day. He took action that acknowledged complexity and sought to grapple with it. His action tried to avoid dividing the patient into individual professionals' conventional duties, and accepted that many different professional perspectives would contribute to everyone's actions and decisions within their own role.

One aim of this chapter is to encourage everyday team building. My answers to the questions posed by its title are: build your team however and wherever you can, in everything you do. Trying to enhance the quality of what we do means calling effectively on the whole range of services and care that might benefit our patients and service users, and coordinating it so that every element of it works together well.

People who talk to me about team building are often fearful of taking a role in it. They see it as a specialist activity, separated from everyday work in team 'awaydays', based on psychological theories of group relations. These ideas aim to improve group and interpersonal relationships, and people often feel that this work needs to be facilitated by external management consultants, uninvolved in internal team relationships, who have special skills to deal with difficult relationship conflicts that might emerge unexpectedly. Sometimes this is an accurate picture, especially when there had been a major change in the organization, or there are particular problems. However, while I do not neglect group relations team building, I focus on a knowledge management approach to everyday team building, which argues that our work will be happier and more successful if we all pay attention to teamwork all the time as part of our practice. The next two sections of the chapter look at these two alternative approaches to team building.

## Two approaches to team building: (i) group relations

Group relations ideas are very powerful in writing and thinking about teamwork, and they treat teams as human groups. They are based on the view that groups take on a life of their own because they need to create a shared identity and purposes, which may be different from the preferences and concerns of the individual members. Teams are part of organizations, which also place expectations on the group to reflect the agreed or approved identity of the organization. In turn, the organization puts people in roles in the team, organizationally defined identities that again cause them to behave differently from how they would behave in a natural human group. Thus, people often find that groups create tensions between their personal aims and hopes and the ways in which they seem to be expected to behave in the group. Teamwork makes this worse because of the additional tensions imposed by organizational objectives and roles.

I say 'seem to be expected' because, in groups and organizations, there are several people involved, representing a range of interests and concerns. This often means that it is unclear what is expected of us and the extent to which it clashes with personal needs and wishes. Team building in a group relations perspective assumes that these tensions and conflicts may sometimes need to be exposed in order to be made clear and dealt with. Exposure of uncertainties and hidden feelings is worrying for people because they do not always know what other people may think of them, and it may lead to relationship difficulties that may cause problems in their future work as part of the team. It may also raise emotions and interpersonal conflicts that are hard to deal with. This is why skilled facilitation from outside the relationships within the team or group seems to be necessary, and also gives the people involved greater confidence that difficulties can be tackled.

The traditional view of group relations team building is developmental, i.e. it sees the purpose of team building as to help a group of people work together *as a group*. Many manuals of team building practice, therefore, emphasize activities to enhance group identity and interaction. A well-known example is Tuckman's (1965, Tuckman and Jenson, 1977) account of small group development, which is often applied directly to teamwork, for example in West's (2004) and Adair's (1986) widely used practical texts. Based on mainly laboratory research into small groups, this identifies five stages of team development:

- *forming*, in which members deal tentatively with getting to know each other and anxieties about what the group is going to be like
- *storming*, in which members try to assert their understanding of their own role and needs
- *norming*, in which members gain experience of working together and build up norms of shared practice
- *performing*, in which members are able to implement the norms fairly inexplicitly as a matter of course and
- *adjourning*, in which members deal with closure, with major losses in their membership and with changes in functioning.

Lying behind this analysis is the assumption either that teams will naturally progress through these stages, as laboratory groups do, or alternatively that they may become hung up at one stage or another and need to be helped to develop to the next stage. It also assumes that the main purpose of the exercise is to create 'performing' groups, rather than the possible alternatives.

However, it may not be desirable or necessary to create a group at all. I argued (Payne 1982, 2000) that a situational view was often more appropriate. For example, Miller *et al.* (2001) studied a wide range of health care teams and found that a variety of models of practice were used, including a group model, a core and periphery model and a model that involved largely individualistic working. Miller *et al.*'s (2001) research supports Lewis's (1975) proposal that teamwork needs to be appropriate to:

- members' preferences
- the type of work they do and
- the kind of organization they work in, which may be divided into:

  field organizations, which need to support people working away from base, such as a palliative home care team

     multiprofessional contexts, where different professional groups need to be
        brought together, such as a palliative care multiprofessional team
     community networking, where different organizations and people of dif-
        ferent statuses, such as volunteers, community activities, politicians and
        professionals, need to be brought together, such as bereavement and
        carers' services, and
     institutional settings, where service users' lives need to be managed in one
        setting, involving domestic, work, leisure and emotional and personal
        support, such as palliative care in-patient units (Payne 2000).

Members' preferences and the type of work often lead to a range of different practices, all of which might be described as teamwork. A common analogy is the distinction between hockey, tennis and athletics teams. In hockey and similar sports, all team members are on the field together and the teams compete directly to score goals. This is like the team on an in-patient ward, where everyone works with patients on the ward, although they may be called into action at different times. Team building may usefully focus first on the group who are present most of the time, and then on how the 'core' team communicates with and passes work to more peripheral members. There may be conflict with and between patients, carers and their families at a time of particular stress for them, and it is easier for different members of families to get one or the other team member to take sides in family disputes with them. Disputes between a team about a patient or family often reflect, and enable team members to work with, conflicts within the family. For example, a social worker and a ward nurse found themselves arguing about the possibility of a father returning home to be cared for by his daughter: could she cope? would he be neglected? Discussing this, they found that the social worker was receiving the father's accusations of the daughter's neglect, while the daughter was telling the nurses how difficult her father's behaviour was. These were long-standing family disputes about the role of a daughter in caring for a parent.

A different form of teamwork comes from tennis teams; all play the same game, but play in their own matches. This is like the home care team, each clinical nurse specialist (CNS) with her own patients within a shared catchment area. Teamwork is about mutual support for the difficult work that nurses often have to carry out alone, isolated from their colleagues, and finding out about and developing resources for patients in their area. For example, a home care team covering a deprived urban area found that the chance to talk about the severe stresses experienced by families in extreme poverty was an important personal support. This was encouraged by working together on a project to improve palliative care in local nursing homes, by providing training and support for inexperienced and underqualified staff in the homes. This might have been seen as an extra stress, but the different nature of the work, the feeling of making progress and the possibility of working together on this project generated better mutual support in work with individual cases. Another useful support was an agreement that where there were difficulties, nurses would visit families jointly, each taking a share of the work in a particular phase of the case.

The third type of team, athletics teams, all play different sports separately. An example is a multiprofessional team working on a complex care case, incorporating people in primary care and adult social services teams.

An example is given in Box 8.1.

---

**Box 8.1** MULTIPROFESSIONAL TEAMWORKING IN A COMPLEX CASE

---

Joe was diagnosed with motor neurone disease, which progressed quickly, and he was admitted to a nursing home when his wife was unable to care for him at home. He had been a physical education teacher, and was very depressed about the loss of his physical prowess, his home, partner and young son. He rejected personal help and disliked the impersonality of the nursing home. His GP referred him to a hospice home care team.

The clinical nurse specialist (CNS) referred him to the complementary therapist, who provided a course of massage, to help deal with pain and increasing immobility in the upper body. She also reviewed and revised his pain control and other medication regularly, consulting with the palliative care consultant physician. The CNS also referred him to the day unit and the social worker. The day unit offered an opportunity for some social involvements and activity. The day unit nurse keyworker liaised with the physiotherapist and nursing staff at the nursing home, so that their treatment was coordinated with the work at the hospice.

The social worker enabled him to talk about the losses of physical capacity, home and his relationships with his partner and son. The partner's teenage daughter by a previous relationship had had a difficult relationship with him, not unlike many teenage relationships with step-parents, but made worse by his bouts of anger at his frustration with his deteriorating physical condition, which eventually led to a child abuse investigation. At this point, the daughter moved out to stay with her birth father. The investigation made Joe feel like a failure at the relationship, which injured his pride as a teacher, and indeed raised the risk that he would be added to the list of teachers unable to practise because of child protection issues in their lives, making him feel discredited in his profession at the end of his career. Joe's partner's guilt about how her daughter had forced him out of the home; her inability to care for him and how both events had caused the loss of his relationship with her and his son were major focuses of work for the social worker. She also liaised with the local child protection team about the investigation, supporting Joe through the experience, and helped to explain to nursing home and hospice staff about the investigation process.

The day unit arranged for a community artist to work with Joe at the nursing home, making a video about his life as a teacher and in the nursing home, addressed to his son when he grew up. Joe also began to develop relationships with other people in the nursing home through joint meditation with another patient who was interested in this technique; this allowed him to feel more in control of his feelings about his illness and the path his life had taken. The spiritual care team volunteer, supervised by the hospice chaplain, talked to him about how this had been a revelation to this practical man, who rejected religion, but found that he valued group meditation and shared experiences. Together with the work on the video, he experienced a renewal of interest in his life and the future. This allowed the social worker to work on planning with his partner for the future of his son.

---

In this case example, different professionals, from different agencies, and from different parts of the hospice took on different aspects of the work with Joe. They communicated carefully with each other about their work, passing on information that would help another worker, and coordinating what they did when working at the same time in a different way. A difficulty arose with the social worker, who was concerned that the video might conflict with her work with the mother and child. This was sorted out by discussion between the two workers. However, as a consequence, the arts and social work teams agreed to meet to discuss the different roles that they took in helping patients express their life stories. This took place in a regular multiprofessional case review meeting, set up to examine the principles behind difficulties that arose in particular cases.

The fact that there are these different types of team responding to different situations suggests that a group's development is not always the main priority in team building. This brings me to my second alternative approach: knowledge management.

## Two approaches to team building: (ii) knowledge management

A situational view of team building requires a different approach to group relations team building, because building better interpersonal and group relations does not respond to a team's need to analyse and decide how to build their preferences, type of work and organization into a suitable form of teamwork. Knowledge management focuses on how we deal with professional or disciplinary knowledge. It does not deny that interpersonal issues may be a factor in teamwork, but it gives priority to doing a good job in the task that the team is formed to do; the task defines team members' identities. There may be personal relationship difficulties, but knowledge management argues that we are united by the task and can put the interpersonal on one side.

The traditional assumption about multiprofessional work has been that we should be clear about and be able to represent the role of our profession in multiprofessional work and negotiations about it. Another traditional assumption is that a profession comes from the knowledge and skills that particularly define that profession. However, much knowledge is shared, and it is perhaps more useful to see the shared knowledge as mountainous country, in which each profession concentrates on climbing one or two peaks of knowledge. They leave other professions to concentrate elsewhere, but with a general awareness of the overall map of the country in which we all operate.

Knowledge management argues that we do not arrive at multiprofessional meetings wearing a professional badge. Rather, we join with colleagues in trying to deal with a complex human situation. Our shared work should focus on the knowledge we are using together, applied to the patient we are working with, rather than organizational or professional divisions. In a team, therefore, our task is to reveal the various aspects of knowledge and skill that people bring to the situation, apply it to the patient, or service user—not all service users are patients; they are often carers or relatives of patients. The task of leadership in the team is to allow different aspects of knowledge to come forward, be expressed and used collectively.

The approach to team building here is to allow team members to bring the particular knowledge and skills that they have together and express and use them to complete the task. They will have their own specialist tasks to complete, and these must be respected, but this individual work should be brought together to complete a shared task (Opie 2003). They come as people; their personal identity embodies or incorporates the knowledge and skill that their profession gives them and also their own personality, style and attitudes.

This has eventual consequences for relationships, however, because successful task completion is a process of shared learning. Team members can use this process to move closer together personally, to gain a better understanding of what each can offer and, through understanding, value all the different contributions more highly. In this way, they come to embody or incorporate in themselves the shared learning of the team; they become a 'community of practice' (Wenger 1998). Communities of practice build up their approach to their work through incorporating their shared learning into their members' way of practising and therefore into their professional identities. A chaplain, doctor, nurse or social worker brings their professional identity, their specialist identity as a palliative care worker, their organizational identity as a health care worker, as a hospice or a palliative care team worker and a community of practice identity that knows how to implement all those more general identities in this particular palliative care team.

## Research evidence on team building

The extensive review of evidence carried out for the UK National Institute for Health and Clinical Excellence (NICE) (Gysels and Higginson, 2004: 215) found that:

The evidence (grade Ia, Ia[sic], and below) strongly supports specialist palliative care teams working in home, hospitals and in-patient units or hospices as a means to improve outcomes for cancer patients, such as in pain, symptom control and satisfaction, and in improving care more widely. The benefit has been demonstrated quantitatively and qualitatively, in studies and in systematic reviews of these.

Given the variety of interventions within each team, more work is needed to test the specific components of palliative care team activity (for example to compare different types of hospital team or hospice, or to test specific ways of working within their practice), and to discover if a different skill mix or interventions performed by the team, are more effective than each other.

This answers one basic question: it is clear that in palliative care, working as part of a team is more effective than not doing so. However, as research findings often do, this raises more questions because it is much less clear who would be in the team and what their special knowledge and understanding would be. It is also unclear how to improve the functioning of a team. This research does not tell us much about what is effective in team building, therefore.

Arising from the limitations of the research findings, therefore, it is useful to ask three questions about:

- the special aspects of palliative care to focus on in team building
- the aims of palliative care team building
- the practical implementation of team building activities.

The next three sections address these issues.

## Team building and palliative care

Palliative care raises three main issues for team building. First, it has a holistic philosophy, so it tries to integrate a range of complex areas of human functioning including at least physical, psychological, social and spiritual aspects of humanity. Other possible areas that palliative care teams draw on are legal, ethical, organizational and policy knowledge. All these areas of knowledge are also interpreted from different points of view. For example, social workers are the only profession involved in health care organizations trained primarily in the social sciences (CSIP 2005), while chaplains primarily start from theological knowledge. Both groups are likely to have different priorities from professions trained primarily in biomedical knowledge. Knowledge management means coming to a view about how we incorporate these different knowledges and views of knowledge within a shared-knowledge environment.

Therefore, the second team building issue for palliative care is the fact that it is multiprofessional, because it seeks to coordinate a number of professional groups to respond to human complexity. The third point is that it is specialist, so it must integrate its work with a range of non-specialized aspects of health and social care.

The research reviewed by Gysels and Higginson (2004) refers to hospital palliative care teams, hospice in-patient units and home care teams. There is also evidence about general palliative care undertaken in primary care; all of these sites of palliative care practice benefit from multiprofessional teamwork, and therefore team members would potentially benefit from team building.

In addition to the need to create effective teamwork within each service, connections have to be made between different aspects of palliative care, to facilitate joint work across organizational boundaries. Palliative care is a specialist service and, therefore, is at a tertiary level of health care provision, so that interaction with primary health care and with secondary health provision, such as hospitals, has to be organized. Vertical integration means looking at connections with colleagues in primary and secondary care. Horizontal integration means looking at links with specialist colleagues concerned with tertiary palliative care and cancer services. However, this distinction has no relevance to many of the non-health care elements of the service. A hospice chaplain, for example, or a social worker does not see their colleagues in other services as part of some hierarchy of specialization, but rather as having different roles in a complex system of services. The health care structure does not seem relevant to these other networks.

Knowledge and understanding cannot be assumed in any part of these structures. People in primary care or social care and in community roles such as a parish priest may be more familiar with the range of resources in a particular community and interactions between local services than the specialist palliative care physician, nurse and social worker. The specialist palliative care professional often assumes a point of view that openness about death and dying is desirable. The need for this may be less clear to other professionals. For example, a palliative care team was helping Mrs Rees, a middle-aged woman dying of cancer, who had three daughters, one of whom, Jean, had learning disabilities and was living in supported housing. Jean's adult social services carers thought that it was inappropriate to discuss Mrs Rees's impending death with Jean, taking the view that this is also how they would have treated a child who was unable to appreciate all the implications of the death. The palliative care social worker persuaded them that openness was desirable, to enable Jean at least to say goodbye to her mother, and to help the bereavement process. This openness then led to Jean wanting to help Mrs Rees; usually her mother had been Jean's helper and she wanted to repay this. Again, social services staff felt this was inappropriate for a dependant woman with learning disabilities. However, it proved possible to devise some activities for Mrs Rees and Jean to take part in together, including preparing a memory box for Jean to remember Mrs Rees after her death.

It is, therefore, an important aspect of team building to build links across boundaries. This is often usefully done as an aspect of internal team building. The palliative care team can jointly identify the links that need to be made, then agree who will take responsibility for each one. Team members can then reach out and draw in useful contacts in service networks that are particularly relevant to them. In Jean's case, for example, it was the social worker in the palliative care team who was thought best able to communicate with adult social care staff.

## Team building aims

Before embarking on team building, we should ask some basic questions about our aims, both ultimate objectives and the aims of team building. The first question to ask is: are there alternatives to teamwork and team building? Among the possibilities are:

- Changing organizational policies, structures and strategies so that better coordination is possible
- Setting up systems for referring, delegating or passing work to the best people to deal with it
- Having a keyworker scheme in which the most appropriate professional is chosen to do most of the work with a particular patient, calling on others as required
- Improving professional qualifying education and continuing professional development to improve coordination
- Using consultation or training in specific cases to allow people to undertake work that is not in their usual remit
- Setting up procedures to ensure that work is coordinated effectively
- Reducing professional specialization, so that more people could undertake a wider range of activities—a key aspect of interdisciplinary teamwork.

Each of these possibilities might be useful in some circumstances, others in other circumstances, none excludes the others and some of them are particular strategies of working together, rather than alternatives to multiprofessional teamwork.

The NHS team effectiveness study (Borrill *et al.* 2001) of 500 teams in many different settings, although not in palliative care, suggests some possible overall aims of team building, since four main characteristics of a team were found to be more effective in achieving successful outcomes and good mental health for team members. These were:

- clarity about objectives, achieved through good leadership
- high levels of participation
- high commitment to quality
- high commitment to innovation.

Team building can usefully focus on enhancing teamwork in each of these areas.

A second set of questions about team building is concerned with how explicit team building should be, and who should be involved in it. Does it happen naturally if people work together? Organizing services is a behind-the-scenes activity. Should it be brought into the limelight of work with patients? If not, a crucial element of the service might be unclear to patients, carers and families. On the other hand, patients might expect the professionals to get on with it, and prefer not to be involved. Do patients, their carers and families know that palliative care is provided in multiprofessional teams? Should they care? Such questions are important because improving teamwork costs effort, time and money, and managers, professionals and service users might all reasonably ask if their involvement in team building really does contribute to better provision of the service. A specialist, holistic, multiprofessional practice may not appear obviously desirable to the service user. Usually, they are accustomed to a simpler form of professional response. They go to their general practitioner, get a prescription or are referred to a practice nurse. They may be visited by a district nurse or be referred to the adult social services of the local authority. Therefore, an important aspect of team development may be including the patient, their family and carers in the work of the team, so that they understand why the team works in this way. To do so, the team will need to be clear about its aims and ways of working, so that they can explain and involve service users in it (see Chapter 4 of this volume).

Answering such fundamental questions about our aims is perhaps best reserved for the conceptual and evaluation chapters. However, team building is a way of helping professionals and the people they serve make choices. Examining the possibilities in this way allows us to identify how we might both undertake and evaluate teamwork and team building as a contribution to palliative care in particular teams, rather than trying to assert that a particular form of teamwork is always right for every team.

## Team building practicalities

Does 'team building' improve teamwork? The idea of 'team building' assumes that we know what a good team is and that we can start from some foundation of 'non-team' or 'poor-team', which we can also identify, and construct from it a 'good-team'. By stressing everyday team building, I have emphasized:

- everybody's responsibility to build teamwork in everything that they do
- the responsibility of team meetings to include team issues in their work.

The difficulty with these tasks is ensuring that we are consistent in taking up these responsibilities. The next two sections examine various ways in which we can work in these issues, first on an everyday basis, and secondly as part of the team's meetings.

## Everyday team building

A consistent pattern of inclusion of teamwork helps with this, for example by looking at a typical sequence of work in a case. Table 8.1 suggests some of the people and groups that might be involved at assessment, planning and review stages of a case. Another approach may also be useful to identify particular aspects of a case that particularly require coordination: admission, assessment and discharge may be important points for more detailed thinking about who should be involved.

Another aspect of everyday team building is the attitude we take to issues when they arise. In teamwork, it is usually helpful not to act in a defensive or critical way. A useful approach is first to try to set clear arrangements within the team:

- agree in the team some general rules of behaviour towards each other, especially where there are strong differences in power and status
- agree when and where difficult issues should be resolved and hold these meetings consistently
- identify and try to resolve uncertainties and barriers to communication or the flow of work (e.g. delays because of part-time working, or because people are in a different building)
- give priority to sorting out problems where people have to deal with each other frequently or where there is a history of conflict over an issue or between particular people (Payne 2000).

Within these agreed guidelines, the team should have agreed rules for dealing with issues that may raise conflict. The following may be helpful:

- realize that if you are anxious or uncertain about raising an issue, it needs to be seen as one that might cause potential conflict
- focus on issues not personalities

**Table 8.1** Team building tasks in a cycle of practice

| Cycle of practice | Teambuilding tasks: consider | Inclusion |
|---|---|---|
| 1. Referral/assessment | Other agencies involved | Patient, family members, carers, people in local community, specialized/local voluntary organizations. |
| | Other professionals | |
| | Potential involvements | |
| 2. Planning and management of patient's care | Agencies involved in plan | Patients, family members, carers, local community members, volunteers, voluntary organizations with a role or excluded. |
| | Professionals involved in plan | |
| | Agencies and professionals excluded | |
| | Agencies with risk/protection role | |
| 3. Reviews | Agencies and professionals involved in plan | As above, especially, complainants, who people who were dissatisfied, people who were difficult. |
| | Agencies with a risk/protection role | |
| | Research/evaluation/audit | |

- identify several alternative options for resolution rather than asking for one absolute response to your issue
- work collaboratively to identify useful aims, rather than trying to say 'what we must do is . . . '
- make decision making explicitly fair by listening to points of view and being open about keeping a balance (Payne 2000).

An example is the way in which a social work qualifying student raised an issue. She had experience in mental health care and had built up a relationship with a patient, Mrs Amin, who occupied a single room on the ward. Mrs Amin had a history of mental illness and was suspicious of the motives of nursing staff and doctors, based on previous experience in a mental hospital. She was also very anxious, and felt that nursing staff did not respond to her need for support. This was probably realistic, because a multiprofessional meeting discussed how she had formed the habit of using the call button more frequently than nurses thought necessary. It was agreed that the dosage of tranquillizing drugs prescribed for her would be increased.

After the meeting, the student thought about the discussion, and found herself being concerned that the patient's medication was being used as a restraining measure, rather than considering alternative ways of dealing with Mrs Amin's anxieties. It seemed to her that the decision was made for the convenience of the nurses and the efficient running of the ward, rather than respecting Mrs Amin's need for reassurance and support. Eventually, she went to see Mrs Amin's primary nurse, or keyworker. They had a discussion about the student's concerns. The possibility that the decision about medication could be seen as potentially oppressive had not occurred to the nurse; she had seen the discussion as being about appropriate medication for a distressed patient. She talked about the process by which doctors prescribed medication for administration within their guidelines by nurses' discretion, and how she perceived the discussion as concerned with gaining guidance about appropriate situations in which to use the prescribed medication and appropriate levels of medication for the patient's needs.

In this multiprofessional situation, there are different types of knowledge in play, each of which has different sources. Among these types of knowledge are:

- the student's knowledge about Mrs Amin's personal responses and attitudes, gained from the student's interpersonal relationship with her
- the medical and nursing team's knowledge about the conventions of prescription and administration of medicines
- the student's knowledge of mental health services, and their particular concerns for human rights, drawn from past experience, which may be undervalued by the student and the team because it comes from prequalification experience, because mental health work is in some ways

distant from the focus of palliative care and because it appears to conflict with the conventions of this present setting

- the student's understanding of the social work role as conferring responsibility for advocacy for patients, even against colleagues, which may lead to fears of team members misunderstanding her attitude and collegiality and may, ultimately, place the assessment of her achievement on placement at risk.

There are a number of points to be made about how these types of knowledge interact. First, only some of the uncertainties arise from specifically professional knowledge, primarily the understanding about medication. Other knowledge comes from past experience and particular knowledge about service users drawn from different sources, at varying distances from the present setting, and with varying levels of credibility. The type of knowledge that may have credibility may vary with different situations. The team members here, because they followed many of the rules set out above in dealing with each other, avoided a conflict situation, and instead worked together to share understanding from these different types of knowledge.

However, a hidden professional knowledge issue arises around advocacy. The international definition of social work (IFSW 2000) regards social justice as one of two primary professional roles, alongside helping individuals solve problems in their lives. This involves equalizing relationships between disadvantaged service users and powerful individuals and institutions. So social workers partly conceive their task as to be to change social and institutional relationships, such as nursing and medical attitudes: that is why it is *social* work. The advocacy role in nursing and medicine is more concerned with responding to unrecognized needs in individual patients, in particular when organizational priorities may clash with patients' needs (e.g. NMC 2004).

Secondly, there is a question of expertise. Doctors and nurses are primarily responsible for prescription and administration of medication, and have pursued this expertise with research and practice rigour. Other forms of expertise may be more broadly held. A common issue in team working is the different perceptions held about each other's role, competence and practice. For example, all team members will have expertise in drawing out patients' concerns and wishes. However, as in this case, members often pick up different issues because of their role or their personal style of work. The relatively powerless role of the student, and the student's history of advocacy in the mental health system perhaps allowed her to empathize with Mrs Amin in such a way as to draw out a particular set of concerns that would not have come out with a busy practical nurse or an apparently authoritative doctor. A spiritual care team member may approach a patient reflectively, and with the right patient may receive communications about issues in the patient's life different from those received by people with a clear health or social care role.

**Table 8.2** Issues for team building work

| Team building issues | Questions you can answer | Things you can do |
| --- | --- | --- |
| Individual development | How do individuals want to develop?<br>What individual development does the team need? | Appraisal<br>Career planning<br><br>Confidence building<br>Skill development<br>Knowledge building |
| Strategic development | Team working **vision**: what kind of team do we want to achieve? | Write a press release<br><br>Draw a coat of arms |
| | Team working **mission**: how do we want to work together? | Team motto<br><br>Rules of behaviour |
| Work flow | How do we get work and how does it pass through and leave the team? | Referrals audit (suppliers)<br><br>Handover audit<br>Forms audit<br>Ward round/case conference audit |
| Communication | What kinds of communication do we use, with whom? | Goldfish bowl, external feedback, audio/video, counting who says what, gender/ethnicity |
| Task differentiation | What skills do we need? | Skills audit; defining skills for different professions |
| Role integration: | How can we build sensible roles? | Boundary-drawing, interlocking circles; concentric circles |
| Problem solving | What teamwork problems do we want | Problems audit; review of difficult cases to resolve? |

*Source*: Payne (2000); West (2004).

These are not only issues of the professional role or the personal style of the professional, but are about the interaction of role and style with the patient's interests and concerns. Some patients will be able to talk about some things with most team members; others may reserve a particular communication for a particular member. One of the reasons for multiprofessional teamwork is to take advantage of these differences to gain a more rounded picture of and respond to a wider range of issues.

To summarize this discussion of everyday team building, I have argued that it requires consistent attention to teamwork as part of daily practice, compliance with appropriate team rules about raising and dealing with contentious issues and a focus on understanding the different types of knowledge raised by situations in which teamwork issues arise. I have also noted that this involves not only the practitioner's role and personal style, but the interaction of these with the service user's views and preferences.

## Team building in team meetings

Teams may strengthen team building behaviour in everyday practice by focusing regularly on team building in meetings and joint activities. This does not exclude special team building events, but suggests that frequent review of team functioning is an important part of everyday shared activity. This may be done in:

- regular case discussion including team functioning
- after-event reviews when a particularly significant event or error has occurred
- reviews when communication or decision making has been difficult.

Everyday team meetings can be a site for such activities; it may be useful to schedule a short part of every team meeting for work on team building. Table 8.2 identifies issues that it may be useful to examine periodically. The team can use these topic areas, and others it identifies itself, as the basis for a regular cycle of team building work.

This can be done as part of ordinary structured discussions, by people presenting papers, leading discussions, discussing relevant journal articles or case reviews. However, team building often uses structured discussion techniques. Some of the most common are set out in Table 8.3, which also includes some

**Table 8.3** Standard team building techniques

| Exercise name | Description | Example |
|---|---|---|
| Boxing | Write things down, put it in an envelope until the end; check whether you have achieved it | One team objective, one personal objective for a team day (say in advance if it will be shared at the end or kept private) |
| Icebreaking | Initial exercise to focus on team outside current concerns. | List team members; draw map of team 'territory' (e.g. a ward) and put people where you are likely to find them; discuss the outcomes |
| Rounds | Each person says one thing about a topic; end on a positive, everyone must say something | Say something you value about the contribution of the person on your right. |
| Snowballing | Discuss topic in pairs, take results to a four, take agreed outcomes to team | Training needs. |
| Ideas blizzard | Define issue, set time limit for everyone to shout out ideas (or do rounds); write everything up, then *filter* ideas to make a plan | How can we do something difficult? Competences for the tasks that we undertake? Training needs. |
| Scaling | List ideas, problems; everyone scales 1–5 how useful/serious they are; total and average then discuss results | Good for assessing how well are we doing? How well are we working together? |
| Forcefield analysis | A line down the middle of a page represents a possible outcome; arrows from the left are things which push us towards the outcome, arrows from the right prevent us from reaching it; scale the strength of the forces | Identifying the pros and cons of an innovation; targeting particular issues that stand in the way and that can push an innovation through. |
| Reframing | List problems and issues; for each one define at least one positive side; assess the reality of the positives | Good for problem solving; can be used with snowballing and ideas blizzard. |

*Source*: Payne (2000) with additions.

comment on topics that can usefully be explored using them. Many of these can be combined, as the example on reframing suggests.

An important aspect of palliative care teams is support in response to the particular emotional stresses of death and dying. It is important not to exaggerate the stresses of palliative care: teams involved with child protection, or with *in vitro* fertilization, or adolescent mental health also deal with difficult behaviour and life transitions evoking emotional responses and family reactions that everyone involved finds difficult. However, this does not deny the importance of developing support as an aspect of team building. West (2004, pp. 158–63) identifies three different aspects of support in teamwork:

- social support, which he further differentiates as:

  emotional support,
  informational support,
  instrumental support and
  appraisal support;

- social climate
- support for team member growth and development.

In this paragraph, I explain a little further. Emotional support means being an active, open listener when another team member has experienced strong emotions. It involves stopping what you are doing and listening to the team member's story of what happened, and being prepared to accept the emotional reaction to it; perhaps the colleague is tearful about a child who has just understood that his father is dying, or frightened by a large, aggressive husband angry at some apparently minor failing in the care of his wife, or relieved when a difficult conversation about discharge from the hospice has gone well. Informational support means being prepared to share information about how you did something, or that will help a colleague achieve something, and not expecting credit or thanks. Signs that this might be important are where the colleague seems stressed, or has just experienced a difficult situation—it is easy to forget what procedure to follow next. Instrumental support means seeing that a colleague has a pile of work, and offering to take over some of her phone calls. Appraisal support means being prepared to help a colleague talk through and look at the alternative interpretations of a difficult situation.

It seems that doing these things is a product more of personality rather than organization: how can we build such support into the organization? There are three approaches:

- Being explicit about these forms of support and that they are expected in the team. Direct teaching, using examples, makes people aware of what they can do.
- Reinforcing supportive behaviour when it happens. People should not expect thanks, but it encourages them when they receive it. A team leader

should take the main responsibility, but anyone who notices positive support should mention it and say how helpful it was.
- Encouraging a social climate in which people give priority to sharing and support as part of what they do, and avoid seeming rushed. Being in a rush is being unavailable to others.

This leads us to promoting an appropriate social climate. Baumeister and Leary (1995, cited by West 2004, p. 155) suggest that important aspects of the effective work relationships include:

- frequent interaction
- sense of stability and continuity
- mutual support and concern
- freedom from chronic conflict.

The importance of frequent interaction is borne out in the NHS team effectiveness study (Borrill *et al.* 2001) summarized above. High participation meant meeting once a week or more.

Although we talk about teams as entities, teams are made up of individuals. We therefore have to think about how team building connects with individual development. Team building may interrupt or conflict with personal development of team members, it may support it or it may be irrelevant to it. If it interrupts or conflicts with the individual's development, there is at least a risk, and I would say a high probability, that teamwork will be obstructed. Individuals are altruistic and value others' personal development, but they also pay attention to their own work satisfaction. Groups of workers who are sometimes marginalized, such as women in male-dominated organizations, or men in female-dominated organizations, or people from minority ethnic groups need particular help. Based on working with women, McDougall (1996) suggests five strategies for potentially disadvantaged groups: (1) explicit career planning as part of the team's work; (2) confidence building, so that people are encouraged to believe in their capacity and contribution; (3) assertiveness skills, to help people in a minority or in a junior position make contributions; (4) skill development in organizational politics; and (5) stress management skills.

One difficulty in promoting individual development where there is stability of staff (so that people get stuck in the same role, or a small team, where there is little opportunity for variety or developing new skills) is to plan in the team for everyone to develop their skills through job enrichment techniques. These would include the following.

- Increasing autonomy and achievement, by finding ways of giving people more control over how they plan and do their work, and by giving them opportunities to report back on conferences, journal articles or other professional development activities of interest to the rest of the team.

- Identifying activities that would enable people to finish a particular project regularly, by, for example, working out clear agreements about signposts in the work that patients and workers can identify and feel a sense of achievement for getting there. We can also identify particular parts of a job that are new or more challenging.
- Rotation allows teams to rotate routine or regular tasks, so that everyone has a chance of trying something new and the tedium is shared out.

Summarizing the discussion of team-based team building, I have discussed areas that may fruitfully be addressed, and typical regular activities that may enable teams to do so. I have also drawn attention to the importance of maintaining support as an aspect of teamwork and to responding to individual development needs within a team context.

## Conclusion

In this chapter, I have identified two approaches to team building: a group relations approach, which sees team building as concerned with improving interpersonal and group relations, and a knowledge management approach which seeks to include and understand the range of knowledge, skills and values embodied in the persons of team members. While not excluding team 'awaydays' as a site of team building, I have emphasized the value of everyday actions, in which people cooperate to understand their various contributions and build a shared understanding of their community of practice.

Palliative care, by trying to respond holistically to its patients, their families and carers, requires a multiprofessional approach to develop better relationships within the palliative care team. To integrate its specialist service with primary and secondary care provision, team members also need to plan to reach out and draw in resources from the wider care and community networks that they are in touch with.

Within the team, developing and following rules about how to raise difficult issues, different types of knowledge and how these interact with the service user's perspectives are important aspects of everyday team building. The team provides a context to enable everyday team building to take place, by developing regular review of teamwork and joint activities, maintaining interpersonal support and an appropriate social climate and responding to individual development needs, especially where some team members may be less powerful or have less social status than others. In this context, addressing the needs of women and people from minority ethnic groups may require careful attention.

## References

Adair J (1986). *Effective Teambuilding*. Pan, London.

Baumeister RF and Leary MR (1995). The need to belong . . .' *Psychological Bulletin* **117**, 497–429.

Borrill CS, Carletta J, Carter AJ, Dawson JF, Garrod S, Rees A, Richards A, Shapiro D and West MA (2001). *The Effectiveness of Health Care Teams in the National Health Service*. http://homepages.inf.ed.ac.uk/jeanc/DOH-final-report.pdf

CSIP (2005). *The Social Work Contribution to Mental Health Services: The Future Direction*. Care Services Improvement Partnership, National Institute for Mental Health in England, London.

Gysels M and Higginson I (2004). *Improving Supportive and Palliative Care for Adults with Cancer: Research Evidence*. National Institute for Clinical Excellence, London.

IFSW (2000). *International Federation of Social Workers: Definition of Social Work*. http://www.ifsw.org/Publications/4.6e.pub.html.

Lewis JW (1975). Management team development: will it work for you? *Personnel* **52** (July–August), 11–25.

McDougall M (1996). Using human resources development to progress women into management. In: Briley S, ed. *Women in the Workforce: Human Resource Development Strategies into the Next Century*. HMSO, Edinburgh, pp. 14–22.

Miller C, Freeman M and Ross N (2001). *Interprofessional Practice in Health and Social Care: Challenging the Shared Learning Agenda*. Arnold, London.

NMC (2004). *The NMC Code of Professional Conduct: Standards for Conduct, Performance and Ethics: Protecting the Public Through Professional Standards*. Nursing and Midwifery Council, London.

Opie A (2003). *Thinking Teams/Thinking Clients: Knowledge-based Teamwork*. Columbia University Press, New York.

Payne M (1982). *Working in Teams*. Macmillan, Basingstoke, UK.

Payne M (2000). *Teamwork in Multiprofessional Care*. Macmillan. Basingstoke, UK.

Tuckman RW (1965). Developmental sequence in small groups. *Psychological Bulletin* **63**, 384–399.

Tuckman B and Jensen M (1977). Stages of small-group development revisited. *Group and Organisation Studies* **2**, 419–427.

Wenger E (1998). *Communities of Practice: Learning, Meaning and Identity*. Cambridge University Press, Cambridge.

West MA (2004). *Effective Teamwork: Practical Lessons from Organizational Research*. BPS Blackwell, Oxford.

# 9

# Communication—an essential tool for team hygiene

*Ian Maddocks*

## Introduction

We know about teams. When we were children, we were urged to participate in team sports, not only for physical exercise but also as a learning experience, exposing us to new relationships, preparing us for opportunities of cooperation and encouraging a form of morality called 'team spirit', a forerunner to patriotism.

Teams accomplish tasks in ways that individuals cannot; the combined efforts of several exceed the sum of contributions acting separately. If we are old enough to have studied Latin, we may once have translated the story of the Roman father who showed his sons how several sticks held together cannot be broken, yet individually they snap easily. Sport provides a common illustration of how teams work, and one characteristic is a common goal; another is diversity of roles and specialization. In football, netball, cricket or baseball, you may show promise as a forward, a back or a goalie, a bowler (pitcher) or a batsman (striker). On the other hand, in a rowing eight, each rower's task of pulling on an oar is almost exactly the same, and the key to success is close coordination, timing exactly the entry of the blades into the water.

During the Athens Olympic Games, an Australian female eight failed to gain a place because one rower stopped rowing in the final stages of the race. She explained later that she felt she had given her all and had no more to give, so she stopped. The consternation and disappointment of her fellow oarswomen was obvious; their comments were not uniformly sympathetic and the discussions that ensued through the Australian media were mostly very critical. She had 'let the team down'. It seemed unlikely that she would be selected for membership of such a crew thereafter. 'Team spirit' puts the task of the team ahead of any individual concern, and all team members need to be seen to be 'pulling their weight'.

## Teamwork in health care

Modern health care is increasingly complex, and no single individual can be competent in all its necessary aspects. It requires the simultaneous intervention of multiple specialist components. Collaborative teamwork is promoted as offering an ideal of comprehensive, seamless service. That ideal may not be easily attained. Institutional health care organizations have traditionally been hierarchical, dominated by male doctors. Although that old male culture is being steadily eroded by the newer culture of the multidisciplinary and gender-equal team, the physician still tends to lead in most circumstances. Each team member will endeavour to provide a contribution to an appropriate professional standard, but assessment of that contribution will rarely include how effectively collaboration with others has been achieved. Demarcation disputes are not uncommon when workers from different professions are asked to help manage the same patient.

Some health team workers seem to take to heart the comment of the old neighbour in Robert Frost's poem, *'Mending Wall'*: 'Good fences make good neighbours', and maintain good working relationships by keeping each other at arm's length.

## Teamwork expected in palliative care

Palliative care is as broad and complex in its professional scope as any other discipline in health care. It is practised in acute hospitals, aged care, community and home care settings, and in specialized hospice programmes. It encompasses internal medicine, pain management, nursing, oncology and radiotherapy, psychology, pharmacy, physiotherapy, occupational therapy, social work, pastoral care, complementary therapy, bereavement counselling, to name only the most prominent contributors. It especially applauds shared care, with different disciplines acting in concert, and seeks to overcome problems of demarcation. It calls for, and expects teamwork to bring those many professional skills together for the welfare of the patient.

## Models of teamwork

There are two major models of multidisciplinary collaboration in health care—the *interactive team* and the *network*. Both require good communication in order to work effectively.

### The interactive team

The interactive team holds its members together in a single structure, often based in a single centre, and all its members will usually be focused on meeting the needs of the one population of patients. We can draw this model as resembling eggs of a different colour or size grouped in a single nest (see Fig. 9.1).

### The multidisciplinary network

In this model, various specialist disciplines, not necessarily based in the one place, but meeting regularly and thoroughly aware of one another, are called upon for their various contributions to the care of a particular patient as and when that contribution is required.

Ahmedzai (2005) has referred to this as a *virtual team*:

Typically, multidisciplinary (or interdisciplinary, or multi-professional) teams operating in cancer, rehabilitation, or similar services arrange to meet physically in a room on a regular—usually weekly—basis, to discuss patients and plan their investigations or care. Supportive care involves the concept of a virtual team composed of collaborating professionals (and in some circumstances, volunteers) from different disciplines, making complementary contributions at all stages of illness, without their having to be present in the same room, or even in the same health care sector. Thus comprehensive supportive care is in reality delivered by a network of individuals, teams and resources.

Where an interdisciplinary team may have a chosen permanent leader or chair or manager, the virtual team may be called into action by any member

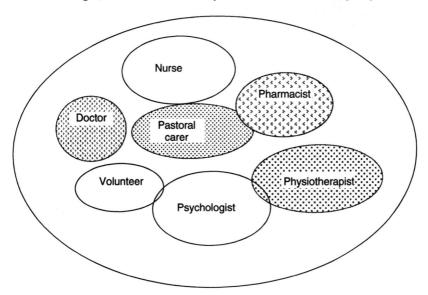

**Fig. 9.1** The interactive, multidisciplinary team.

of the network; it is flexible, opportunistic and less formal. Such a team may be seen in private medicine, where each practitioner has an individual contract with the patient, whereas an interdisciplinary team is funded as a collective, usually with salaried members within a public or charitable system (see Fig. 9.2).

A key to the contribution by any individual to overall team effectiveness is how closely it links with those of other individuals: how well team members read each other's effort and allow for each other, supplement each other's strengths, support each other's weaknesses or deficiencies, maintain the morale of the group, celebrating the spirit of togetherness. A shorthand word for that complex process is 'communication'.

## Communication: a key component in palliative care

Meghani (2004) included effective communication as one of the major characteristics of palliative care; palliative care practitioners are good communicators, at least with their clients. Jack *et al.* (2004) compared insight scores (understanding and acceptance of the reality of their disease) for patients who received intervention from a palliative care team with others who received 'traditional care', and found significantly greater improvement in those in receipt of palliative care support.

Considerable difficulties may present when seeking to explore patient and family understanding and expectations in situations of advanced and terminal illness. Established cultural or family traditions can inhibit direct mention of realities in situations of advanced illness, death and dying. In an increasingly multicultural world, there are barriers founded in differences of language,

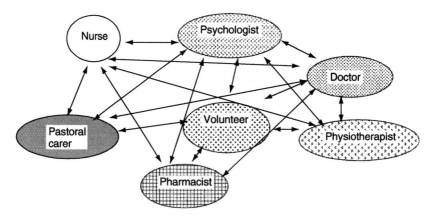

Fig. 9.2 The network.

religion or education. Generational considerations must also be recognized: older clients are often more inhibited than younger persons in revealing their feelings. There are individual traditions of communication style and body language that vary widely. Further, in any particular setting, it may not be clear who has the acknowledged authority to know the facts and make the necessary decisions; it may not necessarily be the patient.

Recognizing these inherent difficulties, palliative care practitioners still have an obligation to decide what to say, and how much. Hallenbeck (2004) suggests two important initial steps in exploring how much to disclose: (1) a statement of respect; and (2) an exploration of the family's prior experience in discussion of serious illness and dying.

A palliative care physician working with aboriginal families in rural Queensland, Australia has described such steps in seeking to explore a difficult clinical case with a senior member of the patient's family. She knew that in aboriginal culture, an individual is often offended by direct eye-to-eye contact; so she asked, 'You have shown me respect by coming to talk with me; how should I show you respect?' The reply was, 'If you really want to know, you should sit on the floor and face away from me'. So she did, adopting for that interview the cultural norm of that aboriginal group.

### Communication within the team

Workers in palliative care may have the reputation of good communication with their patients and families, but do they communicate well with each other? Boyle *et al.* (2004) examined the processes of good communication within a cancer surgery unit. Using the analogy of the rugby team, they highlight key factors for teamwork: pre-match preparation, orientation to the game and the team's particular strengths, sizing up the opposition and exploring creative plays.

### PREPARATION

The preparation for the practice of palliative care commonly involves, nowadays, specific training in psycho-social issues, counselling techniques, and matters of grief and bereavement. It will not as frequently, however, have included a consideration of how to contribute to the smooth functioning of a team. Palliative care has attracted staff who bring a powerful sense of vocation; many see it as a modern form of missionary enterprise. In the early days of development of the discipline, a sense of excitement in being part of a pioneering movement bound its practitioners together in a persuasive enthusiasm. This is not necessarily easy to maintain. One observation of the life of the individual missionary (within the Christian tradition of outreach to distant parts) was that its greatest difficulty often was the need to live in close contact with other missionaries.

## ORIENTATION

Sharing a common understanding of just what is involved in the task of bringing comfort is an essential part of good palliative care practice. Staff seconded from acute medical wards to help in a hospice unit may bring established attitudes that are inappropriate; be disturbed, for example, by the relative lack of interest in the recording of routine observations, or the ready acceptance of alternative forms of practice. Staff need to feel a permission to be responsive rather than prescriptive in their attempts to meet patient and family need. Once oriented, the common rituals of the acute hospital may seem quite unnecessary to the dedicated hospice nurse. A hospice nurse in Adelaide, seconded one weekend to an acute medical unit in another part of the hospital, was asked to weigh all the patients on one side of the ward. *'But its Sunday morning and they are all asleep! Why disturb them to weigh them?'* 'We always weigh the patients on Sunday morning'. *'Well we don't, and I won't do it'.*

## ACKNOWLEDGEMENT OF TEAM STRENGTHS

A major strength for a palliative care team to evolve and protect is the sense of team members looking after each other. Dealing with death on a daily basis can make steady demands on individual resilience. Members of the team need to be aware of each other's vulnerability, and ready to recognize each other's strengths. A pioneering nursing director in Australia used to say that nurses traditionally had been tempted to be 'bitchy', to protect themselves; understandable, perhaps, given the heavy physical and psychological demands laid upon nurses. Within the old hierarchies of nursing, each watched the others, protecting personal rights.

## SIZING UP THE OPPOSITION

Here is the rugby analogy inappropriate? Not necessarily. For many palliative care teams, the opposition is the managerial staff, the administrators of institutions who (it is often felt) fail to understand the special nature of palliative care, and seek to impose routines of reporting and cost control that constrain desirable practice and offer no recognition or applause for work done well. To help members of a clinical team cope with the complexity of modern medical care in the USA, Leonard *et al.* (2004) suggested they need to feel encouraged to speak up and express their concerns, and called for the development of a common language for indicating critical or difficult (unsafe) situations. Similar encouragement may help hospice team members be defended against the oversight of the managers, which Vachon (1987), in an early study of hospice care, described as the greatest source of stress for team members.

EXPLORING CREATIVE PLAYS

Palliative care is an excellent setting for creative clinical intervention, because of the lack of established guidelines for situations that so often are individual and unique. Exploring favourite items in personal experience may encourage more intentional use of music, food brought from a well-known café, a whisky before bed time, a trip to the beach, the theatre or the zoo in a wheelchair. Conventional and unconventional therapies may find an equal place—morphine with meditation, antiemetics and acupuncture, aromatherapy together with corticosteroids, Reike with respiratory support.

## The team meeting—an opportunity for good communication

The multidisciplinary team meeting is where, through opportunity for open exchange and good communication, consensus is achieved concerning attitude, philosophy and management of practice, and specific interventions planned for individual patients and their family members. It is a place for telling the story of one's own patient encounters, and for checking it against the accounts of others. Some staff may wish to recount intimate details gleaned from close personal interactions, if only to demonstrate their excellent rapport. Visiting the home, a nurse may have learnt, for example, of a child born years ago out of wedlock and adopted out, never revealed within the later marriage, and now a source of quiet distress to the dying mother. Skeletons can fall from the cupboard during the closing phase of a life, but need not be proclaimed to the whole team. Leadership should establish an expectation that permission for disclosure of such private information is sought, and that only those team members are informed whose understanding and support is important to that individual patient.

Communication between professionals from different backgrounds may present difficulties if there is inadequate understanding of specialist roles, and impatience with the style and language used. Weissman (2001) has pointed out that when physicians are required to take difficult decisions, non-physician health professionals may perceive them as uncaring or callous, and fail to recognize that such apparent behaviour may represent the outward expression of fears and uncertainties. A team culture will be helpful if it encourages other staff to say not, 'Why is he being so mean?' but rather 'Doctor, this must be quite hard for you'.

Attempts to improve cross-professional understanding have included introduction to each other's disciplines during training (see Chapter 10 of this volume). Fineberg *et al.* (2004) compared the understanding of each other's roles in groups of medical and social work students who either participated in combined training sessions or were given written information. Those who shared the training (which focused on the promotion of professional interaction and the building of mutual trust and respect) showed much better understanding than those who had only written materials, and the difference remained apparent 3 months later.

More could be done to assist the inclusion of the chaplain in the clinical palliative care team. A review of chaplain perceptions in the UK suggested that although they commonly attend multidisciplinary meetings, they often felt like outsiders, rarely called upon by nursing staff, and many felt that they themselves provided spiritual support (Lloyd-Williams *et al.* 2004). 'I doubt if anyone really knows what I do' was the rather sad comment of one chaplain.

### Including non-professionals

A strong volunteer component is a proud characteristic of many palliative care units. Volunteers who offer presence, sitting alongside anxious patients, or provide cups of tea for distressed relatives can have extremely useful insights to offer and should be represented in team exchanges. Spouses or other key family members are often left out of the team discussion when their input could be critical in framing an optimal approach to care (see Chapter 4 of this volume). This can also be of great importance when the treatment and care of the patient raises ethical concerns. Misunderstanding and poor communication can enhance the tension often experienced around ethical decision making.

### What makes a healthy team?

In both models of the team, mentioned earlier, the setting of an agreed goal, and maintaining an agreed process towards the achievement of that goal, will depend on a number of factors. These have been explored in situations as diverse as neonatal care (Miller 2005), aged care (Coogle *et al.* 2005), and accident and emergency wards (Macfarlane *et al.* 2004). The value of a culture of humour, 'extracurricular' activities (coffee breaks, sports, concerts and weekend retreats) and organized counselling programmes is suggested—all of which can contribute to improved communication. The example of clear lines of authority and responsibility, found most obviously in military groups, helps any team establish a cooperative culture, but need not be rigidly hierarchical. Maturity and previous practical experience in the area enhance confidence in an individual's approach to sharing; and training, not only in the content of the discipline, but also in the team process is recommended.

Astudillo and Mendinueta (1996) described exhaustion syndrome as a potential risk for palliative care workers, one destructive of good teamwork. They suggested prevention by early recognition of job stress, the maintenance of good relationships among team members and administrative measures that provide support in addressing difficult matters. Failure of recognition by distant administrators of the special characteristics of palliative care work (flexibility, ability to be creative and unconventional in care approaches, and to respond to unusual demands), and insistence by them on strict adherence to rules (whether concerned with uniforms, time sheets, observation charts or any other of the everyday matters that administrators require) are far more stressful to workers than their daily tasks of caring for dying persons.

## Common issues for either model of team work

Terms used to indicate collaboration in everyday experience may have positive or negative connotations. Hutchins *et al.* (2003) noted the words that might be used in referring to collaboration include *association, cooperation, consultation* and *partnership*. These represent a favourable view of team working; critics of a team, however, may be using more negative words: *conspiracy, collusion* or *competition*.

### Leadership

How leadership is conceived and practised (whether as occasion demands or as an established function for one person), who undertakes the role of leader, how the leader is chosen, how delegation of authority is achieved and how leadership can be changed may all differ widely and affect the quality of both inter- and intrateam communication (see Chapter 5 of this volume). The most senior or most qualified person within the team may easily assume the role, but unless the role of the leader is clarified, and open discussion occurs about options for team management, there may be simmering discontent, with some team participants judging that the group is dysfunctional but feeling power-less to change it.

In some cultures, an open discussion is readily agreed, and the choice of leader may be resolved harmoniously; not necessarily falling to the senior doctor or remaining with one person indefinitely, but changing regularly. In other cultures, such discussion is more difficult. One Japanese colleague, a psychiatrist, explained the working of his palliative care team: 'At our team meeting we discuss a case. The resident describes the case, the nurse gives her opinion, I give my opinion, then the Professor gives his opinion and that is what we do'.

### Commitment and 'ownership'

Interactive team members readily form an 'in' group and it is sometimes hard for them to recognize when they are not sufficient. Palliative care often recruits individuals with a sense of vocation, from a base in the Christian traditions of mission, altruism and succour for the needy. There is the risk of finding a confidence in a common commitment ('we all share the same faith') and failing to recognize the team's deficiencies, or the times when they need additional help. Incestuous self-satisfaction may make it difficult for a new member of staff to feel part of the team, particularly if that new arrival has some ideas for change or improvement of the service. There may also be an assumption that staff will 'go the extra mile', with latent criticism of those who stick to their hours or the terms of their job statements (or take time off for unexplained reasons, like the unfortunate Olympic oarswoman). Sharing stories, team members will remind each other of the good things being accomplished, but 'a multiplicity of anecdotes is not data', and objective outcomes of the team's activity may be less impressive. Teams need to know their limitations and where to get help (Hull *et al.* 1989).

Webster and Kristjanson (2002) invited long-term workers in palliative care nursing to respond to the question, 'What kept me here?' The answers were along these lines: 'Probably more than anything else a commitment to what we do. To the philosophy of palliative care I think, and to seeing that practically worked out in the lives of our patients and families. That, along with working with a great team of people. I like working with other disciplines. And it's one area where you do work with other disciplines. Where, although it doesn't always succeed, there is a philosophy for multidisciplinary care, holistic care'.

Goodwill and commitment are not in themselves enough, however; continuing learning and research are also basic to good clinical practice.

Within a network team, there will be some members more aware of other parts of the network, and more used to working cooperatively. Family doctors will be used to dealing with community nurses, but specialist doctors less so (Goldschmidt *et al.* 2005). There is a risk of 'ownership' issues intruding and limiting an appropriate gathering of the necessary expertise required for a difficult situation.

### Team size

How big can a team be? Increasing workloads, bringing recruitment of new individuals with different skills, will add to the complexities of management, and require more bureaucratic processes, threatening the intimacy and informal trust readily found in a small stable group. It will also affect communication routines, which must be revised as a team enlarges. Whereas initially every team member may join a weekly meeting discussing individual patients, as size begins to exceed 20 or more staff and >100 patients in the programme, the time required grows and seems an unnecessary duty for many participants. Delegation, and separation of responsibilities to subgroups, will become essential; the use of IT technologies to share decisions across subgroups may work well. The sense of one team must be protected, however, by continuing

efforts to maintain a sense of common team purpose, ensuring prompt introduction and incorporation of new members, making an agreed adjustment of
roles in response to change and inventing new styles of celebration for the
team as a whole and for its individual members.

### Roles and rituals—possible contributors to meaningful communication

Mallet *et al.* (2002) discuss the activity of the palliative care team within the
major hospital as a meeting of two distinct cultures, each with different rituals.
The interest of palliative teams in spiritual care and its simple rituals serves to
counter the excessive objectivism of medicine and helps to maintain a sense of
purpose in care and a search for meaning around the reality of dying.

The two cultures must establish common ground, mutual respect, and a
policy of shared care and seamless oversight based in that respect, if the
transfer of a patient from the care of one team to another is not to be interpreted as abandonment.

Within the team, the role of each member needs clear definition. The place
of the physiotherapist, the pharmacist or the chaplain within the team is often
left vague, and the work assigned to them must often be accomplished on
a part-time basis. A physiotherapist, whose work elsewhere calls for active
encouragement in building muscle strength and mobility or enhancing
respiratory function, needs to change approach in bringing to the hospice
ward some gentle massage techniques, lymphoedema care or instruction for
nurses in lifting techniques. Some units have the luxury of a pharmacist to
check all drug orders, and bring medication advice to team meetings; others
use the pharmacist only to restock their cupboards. Particular vocabulary and
jargon attends each specialty, and all team members need to ensure that their
pattern of communication is free from pretentious or arcane expression, and
framed in terms that all members of the team can understand easily.

### Style

Each situation of human exchange has its own elements of style. Many factors
influence the detail of how communication is expressed and exchanged.
Clearly culture plays an important part, but to try to elaborate how ethnicity,
language and history affect style would be an extensive task beyond the scope
of this chapter. Within Western and English-speaking culture, there are wide
variations in style of address, influenced by age, gender, education and particular historical context. Most individuals will alter their style of communication with the social context in which they are placed. They will not use the
same vocabulary or tone of voice in a church as at a football match; and they
will not address an older or respected person in the way they speak to a friend
or a child. When my father was receiving care in a hospice and the staff

commonly addressed him by his Christian name, his granddaughter saw that as disrespectful, 'They shouldn't talk to grandpa like that'.

He himself, in an earlier phase of nursing home care, had noted, 'They speak to me as though I am a child'. Polly Toynbee, in her study of a London hospital found a similar reaction among patients subjected to a familiar mode of address such as, 'Hop up on here, dear'—to someone whose days of 'hopping' were long passed.

Dress has its impact on style also. Thirty years ago, a surgeon at my hospital wrote in the student newspaper deploring the failure of some students to appear properly dressed in their white coats. I responded with an alternative view, suggesting that the white coat created its own barrier between professional and client, something unnecessary and unhelpful. Nowadays, neither students nor staff at that hospital wear white coats (yet communication may not have improved), and white coats are not seen in any of the Australian hospices I visit. Style also comprises body language and volume of speech, details of which we may be unconscious. After leaving an exchange with a difficult bureaucrat, my psychologist companion said to me, 'Are you aware that as you become more angry you sink lower in your chair and your voice becomes softer and softer?' Similarly, a senior nurse noted, after we had left the bedside of a dying patient, 'Your voice dropped into the quiet confiding tone you use when giving bad news'.

Communication within a health care team will have its own traditions and its own style. It is common for relatively black humour to be a medium of exchange. A patient in an oncology unit who responds to therapy less well than hoped, and who remains uncomfortable and persistently complaining, is referred to by her physician as 'my albatross' (shades of the Ancient Mariner). Irreverent descriptions of colleagues or of difficult relatives may relieve team stress, and encourage laughter. However, quiet testimony of moving examples of love and courage can also be aired, and reinforce team solidarity and resolve.

### Techniques for communication

Face-to-face exchange remains the best, and this emphasizes the value of co-location of team members. Much useful exchange happens through chance corridor meetings. Communication also needs to be more intentional and deliberate, in case such chances do not occur. Team meetings are of great value, but take up valuable time. How team exchanges and decisions are recorded is an additional issue.

Urgent contact with the persons who can provide assistance when it is needed is essential for crisis management. Modern technology speeds ahead of imagination, and it is difficult to envisage with any clarity how the incorporation of immediate visual and voice contact using modern video-telephones will change the way we work. There will surely be less excuse for not communicating, but will we be overloaded by irrelevant and unnecessary contact? Wiecha and Pollard (2004) argue that the Internet is a logical platform for supporting interdisciplinary clinical teamwork, because of its synchronous and asynchronous communication capacity and information-gathering and sharing capabilities. However, the plethora of unwelcome and unhelpful E-mail messages many of us now receive is a warning. Also, what is worth recording? Too much indiscriminate data are exhausting and confusing; the unit database rendered unwieldy.

We should not neglect simple paper-based records, particularly those that are kept close to the centre of our interest—the patient. I recall from many years ago, when working in an African paediatric out-patients, that large African mothers would extract from somewhere in the vicinity of their cap-acious bosoms small sheets of paper containing the past medical records of their infants, carefully preserved, never lost, always available. The patient-held record, kept in the home and accessed by doctor, nurse, family and other carers, can be the most valuable tool for community care.

The patient record will not provide a basis for research unless it is designed to be retrieved and its entries added to a central data bank. How this is to be achieved, whether through the transfer of paper or through the wonders of information technology, is an excellent topic for team discussion.

## Conflict

Clashes and conflicts within teams must be anticipated. Palliative care workers often demonstrate great dedication to their work. Strong characters, con-firmed in their sense of vocation, may be uncompromising, sure of their own opinions and practices. Some clashes stem from differences in training and professional viewpoint; others are based on personality, reflecting different personal histories and backgrounds, styles of communication and exchange, individual habits and preferences.

In quite a long experience as a member of a Medical Board, receiving complaints about doctors, I was aware that the great majority of angry com-plaints arose not from surgical error or physician incompetence, but through a failure to establish an open and honest communication between professional and client. Similarly, within the team; unless there is a free sharing, misunder-standings will arise, and hurt and hostility be engendered. Differences may be based in the sense of ownership ('He is "my" patient') or professional jealousy ('Shouldn't you leave the counselling to me?')

Conflicts may also arise in the context of ethical decisions that commonly confront palliative care teams—whether a new clinical presentation should be investigated, and whether it needs potentially curative treatment or simply comfort care. It will be natural for other staff to defer to the expertise of the doctor in many situations, but in others the staff who work more intimately

149

with the patient and family (particularly the nurses) may feel they have a better grasp of the real needs and wishes of the patient than the doctor can achieve in the normally brief medical consultations.

The work of the interactive palliative care team in an in-patient hospice is largely separated from continuing 'curative-type' therapies. Within a network model, however, continuing chemotherapy or radiotherapy for advanced cancer may be expected, and such potentially discomforting treatments can become a point of contention: 'They want to give her more of those awful poisons' from the palliative care worker, or 'He's not ready for you yet' from the oncology team. Similarly, conflict may arise over the place of complementary medicine within the care being offered by the team, particularly if it involves bringing in therapists strange to the other team members, and offering therapies that are not familiar and seem to communicate in a 'foreign' language.

In the areas of policy and administration of a palliative care service, there will not always be agreement about *which* patients should receive priority in admission for palliative care, *when* in the course of the illness a particular individual becomes eligible for palliative care, *where*, for that person, it will best be delivered, or *how* it will be delivered. The way those questions are answered will depend partly on *who* is included in the team discussion.

### Communication with other palliative care teams

When a patient needs to transfer to a different region or to change the site of care (hospital to home, aged care facility to hospice) adequate 'hand-over' is essential. There will also be advantage in regular meetings where members from different teams learn from each other. In the absence of universal guidelines, many palliative care units will have evolved individual ways of managing difficult situations, and sharing methods can benefit everyone. Common problems in advocacy or fundraising may be met most satisfactorily by combined action, and drawing upon members of another team for teaching exercises prevents staleness and repetition.

Contact needs to be maintained also with other clinical teams, to obtain specialist advice, to be known by them for the helpful opinion the team can offer, to educate (enlarging the sometimes narrow perspective of a different specialty) or to participate in teaching undertaken by other disciplines.

## Conclusion

The reputation won by members of palliative care teams for close interaction and cheerful cooperation is well deserved. Some of those characteristics may have been fostered by the sense of being 'special', and pioneering a new discipline, a new social movement. As palliative care enlarges its brief to include care of individuals other than those with advanced cancer, and as it finds a more established place in health care, it may expect to lose some of that sense of being special. We must hope that if it is seen as increasingly 'ordinary', it does not lose those necessary high standards of communication.

## References

Ahmedzai S (2005). The nature of palliation and its contribution to supportive care. In: Ahmedzai SH and Muers MF, ed. *Supportive Care in Respiratory Disease*. Oxford University Press, Oxford, pp. 3–38.

Astudillo W and Mendinueta C (1996). Exhaustion syndrome in palliative care. *Supportive Care in Cancer* **4**, 408–415.

Boyle FM, Robinson E, Heinrich P, and Dunn SM (2004). Cancer: communicating in the team game. *Australian and New Zealand Journal of Surgery* **74**, 477–481.

Coogle CL, Parham IA, Cotter JJ, Welleford EA and Netting FE (2005). A professional development program in geriatric interdisciplinary teamwork: implications for managed care and quality of care. *Journal of Applied Gerontology* **24**, 142–159.

Fineberg IC, Wenger NS and Forrow L (2004). Interdisciplinary education: evaluation of a palliative care training intervention for pre-professionals. *Academic Medicine* **79**, 769–776.

Frost R. (1969). Mending Wall. In: *The Poetry of Robert Frost*. Henry Holt and Company, New York, p. 33.

Goldschmidt D, Groenvold M, Johnsen A, Stomgren A, Krasnil A and Schmidt L (2005). Cooperating with a palliative home-care team: expectations and evauations of GPs and district nurses. *Palliative Medicine* **19**, 241–250.

Hallenbeck JL (2004). Communication across cultures. *Journal of Palliative Medicine* **7**, 477–480.

Hull R, Ellis M and Sargent V (1989). *Teamwork in Palliative Care*. Radcliffe Medical Press, Oxford.

Hutchins S, Hall J and Lovelady B (2003). *Teamwork: A Guide to Successful Collaboration in Health and Social Care*. Speechmark Publishing Ltd, Oxford, pp. 32–33.

Jack B, Hillier V, Williams A and Oldham J (2004). Hospital based palliative care teams improve the insight of cancer patients into their diseases. *Palliative Medicine* **18**, 46–52.

Leonard M, Graham S and Bonacum D (2004). The human factor: the critical importance of effective teamwork and communication in providing safe care. *Quality and Safety in Health Care* **13** (Suppl), 185–190.

Lloyd-Williams M, Wright M, Cobb, M and Shiels C. (2004). A prospective study of the roles, responsibilities and stresses of chaplains working within a hospice. *Palliative Medicine*, **18**, 638–645.

Macfarlane D, Duff EMW and Bailey EY (2004). Coping with occupational stress in an accident and emergency department. *West Indian Medical Journal* **53**, 242–247.

Mallet D, Soyer S, Herbaut A, Daniel M and Prent K (2002). Rituals of the hospital palliative care team. *European Journal of Palliative Care* **9**, 244–246.

Meghani SH (2004). A concept analysis of palliative care in the United States. *Journal of Advanced Nursing* **46**,152–161.

Miller LA (2005). Patient safety and teamwork in perinatal care—resources for clinicians. *Journal of Perinatal and Neonatal Nursing* **19**, 46–51.

Toynbee P (1977). *Hospital.* Hutchinson & Co, London.

Vachon ML (1987). Team stress in palliative/hospice care. *Hospice Journal – Physical, Psychosocial & Pastoral Care of the Dying* **3**, 75–103.

Webster J and Kristjanson LJ. (2002). Long-term palliative care workers: more than a story of endurance. *Journal of Palliative Medicine* **5**, 865–875.

Weissman DE (2001). Managing conflicts at the end of life. *Journal of Palliative Medicine* **4**, 1–3.

Wiecha J and Pollard T (2004). The interdisciplinary health team: chronic care for the future. *Journal of Medical Internet Research* **6**, 113–117.

# 10

# Training in the interdisciplinary environment

*Iain Lawrie and Mari Lloyd-Williams*

## Introduction

Teamwork is integral to palliative care. It's an interdisciplinary entity. It epitomizes the ideal of bringing members of various disciplines together to work in harmony, with a common goal, to provide a 'gold standard' of care. It is a specialty based on multiprofessional, interdisciplinary, transdisciplinary thinking—whatever term one wishes to use—with the central focus being the patient and those close to them, and the emphasis being on quality of life and quality of care. Such standards of excellence, to which every patient is entitled, are only possible where those involved in providing such care are both appropriately knowledgeable and skilled. The acquisition of knowledge and skill, however, does not occur at a single point in one's career. Education and personal growth is a continuum starting at initial basic or undergraduate training and progressing throughout a lifetime in the specialty. The need to keep up to date is demanded by both individual practitioners and their professional regulatory bodies but also, increasingly, by patients—our clients.

Teaching and learning are key elements in both the philosophy and the activity of all those involved in the practice of palliative medicine. Nurses, physicians, physiotherapists, occupational therapists, day care managers, volunteer coordinators, chaplains—all members of the palliative care interdisciplinary team—are in some way involved in either adding to their own knowledge and skills bases or assisting in the development of those of others. Often, usual practice is to concentrate on the education of others, equipping them with both theoretical knowledge and practical skills to introduce a 'palliative care approach' to their own work. Equally important, however, is the continuing education and development of palliative medicine professionals in order that the provisions of high quality care can be continued.

The boundaries that existed between different professional groups have become less distinct over recent years, partly as a result of developments in health care provision (Horsburgh *et al.* 2001). Teamwork is seen as one essential component for effective patient care, the team being both the limited group of professionals working together in a distinct environment and the wider team of, for example, an entire hospital, health authority or national health service. Interdisciplinary training can claim to have originated for many different reasons, such as economic pressures on institutions or fostering a collaborative and more effective working atmosphere. Wherever its beginnings lie, this form of training is now viewed as one of several vehicles for continuing professional development and one that is likely to become increasingly common within health care.

The emergence and development of terms such as multidisciplinary, multiprofessional, interdisciplinary and transdisciplinary is relatively recent, and the associated distinctions and confusion are discussed in Chapter 2. Whether multiprofessional or interdisciplinary is the correct terminology is, in some ways, less important here. What is important is that such an approach to both undergraduate and postgraduate training in health care has been the subject of growing interest over recent years, as there is a belief that it is beneficial to both wider collaboration and within a distinct teamwork environment (Carpenter 1995; Barr and Waterton 1996). The government believes that this approach will in turn help to achieve the core objective of better patient care (Department of Health 2000, 2001).

In this chapter, we shall discuss various elements involved in training that occurs in the palliative care environment that, either through accident or design, often involves individuals from more than one profession or discipline. The intention is not to provide the reader with a recipe for providing interdisciplinary education programmes, but rather to discuss the influences important to such an approach in order that provision can be tailored to individual needs and situations and may, therefore, ultimately prove more effective.

## Adult learning needs and styles

Prior to embarking on a programme of education for any group, especially one involving participants from different professional backgrounds, it is important to consider why individuals wish to learn and, perhaps more vital, *how* they learn. Without consideration of the learning needs and styles of those involved, it may well be impossible to plan and implement education and training effectively. Failure to consider the background from which adults approach learning can lead to poor experiences which, in turn, can give rise to a profound sense of demoralization of both facilitator and learner, and can inhibit further attempts to foster a positive approach to continuing education in the workplace.

The principles of adult learning are outlined in Table 10.1. Adults need to embark on a learning activity with a pre-determined purpose, whether that be simple enjoyment of the subject or, rather more pragmatic, to achieve career advancement or to gain confidence in management of different scenarios they may encounter in their routine work. The concept of voluntary participation in learning is central. In order to participate fully and therefore gain from training, adults must actually *want* to learn to engage effectively in the educational activity. This is also associated with the degree to which the learner views the activity as being relevant to both them and their needs, as they are unlikely to learn if they cannot envisage a situation in which they will be able to apply the knowledge gained or skill acquired.

Preferences for learning methods differ between individuals. As they progress through their careers, individuals develop different styles of working, are employed in various settings and specialize within their own practice, all of which should place emphasis on diversity and produce a wide range of preferences for learning styles (Richmond 1988). Therefore, those planning educational activities should try to avoid 'monotonous uniformity of training activities' (Richmond 1988). Knowles (1973) observed that, as an individual matures, 'his readiness to learn is decreasingly a product of his biological development and academic pressure and is increasingly the product of the development tasks required for the development of his evolving role', i.e. based on perceived and actual needs.

## Strengths and weaknesses of training in an interdisciplinary environment

If one is to accept that the concept of interdisciplinary training within palliative care is both appropriate and desirable, one must also recognize that there are both positive and negative aspects to its use in professional development.

**Table 10.1** Principles of adult learning
(Beard and Hartley, 1984)

Adult learning must be purposeful
Adults must be voluntary participants in learning
Adults require active participation in learning
Adults require clear goals and objectives to be set
Adults need feedback
Adults need to be reflective

Interdisciplinary training is much more than simply getting people from different backgrounds together in the same room. The term 'shared learning' has been used (Horsburgh *et al.* 2001) to emphasize the distinction from 'shared teaching', where the process and aims of the educational activity may not have been fully thought through prior to implementation. Economic pressures often lead to shared teaching activities, where professionals may experience the same educational activity, but may not derive any benefit, i.e. they do not learn. This process is entirely passive and, rather than fostering collaboration between members of different professions, may actually serve to reinforce their differences and increase mistrust, described as 'hostile stereotyping' (McMichael and Gilloran 1984). Shared learning, on the other hand, suggests a successful, effective experience where learners actively participate to achieve pre-determined, relevant and realistic goals which enhance their personal development and, in many areas of health care, improve the service and care provided for patients.

It may be useful to consider the strengths and weakness of training in an interdisciplinary environment from three main perspectives: those of the individual, the team and the organization.

### The individual

For the individual practitioner, such an approach to education can help them recognize that they have a valuable contribution to make, as each team member can bring expertise on a different topic. This can reinforce one's sense of self and, through sharing their discipline's values and culture, affirm their professional identity. It may also serve to increase both personal and professional satisfaction in one's work and allow shared ownership of the development of both the individual and the team. The nature of palliative medicine can be incredibly stressful, not necessarily in terms of workload volume but rather in the physical, psychological and emotional demands it places on those providing care. Interdisciplinary, collaborative training can be a means for colleagues to provide support to each other, through reflective practice, group discussion and as a forum for problem solving. In this way, it can be an adjunct to stress management.

'Hostile stereotyping' (McMichael and Gilloran 1984) has already been mentioned as a potential weakness of this type of educational activity. Where team members do not fully understand or value either the roles of their colleagues or the aspirations of an interdisciplinary training programme, they can be anxious as to the implications for their own practice and place in the team. Should this 'role tension' (Corner 2003) develop, individuals may not feel that they can contribute equally and be supported, and can feel marginalized and excluded. This can result in their contribution to, satisfaction with and sense of ownership of the process being reduced, thus making them feel less valued.

## The team

While the aim of working in health care teams is often to bring about care that is coordinated and effective, the aim of training in teams is to bring together knowledge from the basis of a common learning culture. A team can be an assembly of individuals meeting at a pre-arranged time, or it can be far more dynamic and productive, representing a 'coalition of colleagues' (Farrell *et al.* 2001), which has a shared vision and common goals, as well as an active desire to learn. Training within a team from diverse backgrounds, professionals can begin to explore and understand each other's role within the team, a process that may often be taken for granted in the day-to-day work of an organization. This can be the first step towards more effective team building where roles and responsibilities are shared, and can be the springboard towards truly pooling expertise and sharing the burden of work within the team in order to create a 'combination of skills that no single individual demonstrates alone' (Crawford and Price 2003).

The members of the team being trained, and the relative number of professionals from any given discipline, can contribute both positively and negatively to the effectiveness of an interdisciplinary education programme. Hidden dynamics can exist between both colleagues and professional groups that can adversely affect the success of interdisciplinary learning activities. Corner (2003) observed, 'the more education the team members have, the more prominent and task orientated they are'. Health care has its foundations in a typically hierarchical structure, often with the physician as the 'leader', and palliative medicine may have become 'colonised by an increasingly biomedical and technical approach' (Corner 2003). There is thus the possibility that biomedical ideas, styles and goals may dominate interdisciplinary training and that non-medical participants feel less able to contribute fully.

## The organization

For the organization, the benefits that can be gained from appropriate, well-designed interdisciplinary training are many. Teams become more cohesive and, through a greater understanding of each member's role and expertise, can both share information and complement each other's involvement. This should, in turn, lead to improved patient care and a more effective organization. The analogy of the hand described by Parker (1994) is fitting here: separate digits, whose ability, function and proficiency differ, can achieve more than the sum of the individual digits when they work together. Crawford and Price (2003) described this as, 'when there is some role overlap, resources are actually multiplied and patients can have access to a multi-skilled practitioner who has learned from and been extended by different professions'.

In palliative medicine, challenging scenarios arise that can frustrate the working of the organization, as they have no clear biomedical or social solution. Through using different frameworks for the provision of continuing professional education, of which interdisciplinary training would be an example, the team may find 'new ways of seeing' that can be 'the keys to resolving not only clinical but ethical dilemmas' (Crawford and Price 2003).

While the organization may benefit from the fruits of interdisciplinary training, it may also frustrate its implementation and development. The logistics of permitting members of staff to be available to participate in education sessions, as well as having them in the same location at the same time in the case of larger, dispersed teams, can be challenging in itself and could be seen as a weakness of this approach. An appropriately supportive organizational context—the organization being *explicitly* supportive of interdisciplinary training—is essential for its success and effectiveness.

## Delivering interdisciplinary training in palliative care

The delivery—perhaps a better term would be 'acquisition' to place emphasis on the active participation of the learner, rather than the teacher, being central to the process—of an educational activity can take many forms. However, there are several important stages to consider before addressing the 'how' of programme delivery. While these are each discussed in turn, it should be remembered that in practice each occurs in parallel, and each informs the other stages.

As mentioned earlier, merely gathering a number of individuals from different professional backgrounds together in the same location does not necessarily guarantee that shared understanding will develop (Clark 1993). Four key dimensions to effective interdisciplinary learning have been described, as outlined in Table 10.2 (Parsell and Bligh 1999).

Clear goals, or learning outcomes, are essential to provide direction for the session, for the programme and for participants. Learners must be able to see the relevance of the activity to their work and to their own learning needs. In many instances, it may be more effective to involve participants in the planning process and decision making from the outset, as this can reinforce feelings of ownership and responsibility for learning and can, in turn, ensure relevance. Learning must be structured in order to be effective, with clearly

**Table 10.2** Key dimensions of interprofessional learning (Parsell and Bligh 1999)

Relationships between different professional groups
Collaboration and teamwork
Roles and responsibilities
Benefits to patients, professional practice and personal growth

stated and not overly ambitious learning outcomes planned from the outset. Team goals should be identified at an early stage in order that education sessions can be planned and a logical progression of learning can occur. Early identification of goals also allows for team members to find a common starting point in their existing knowledge from which learning can develop.

The makeup of the team itself should be given careful consideration. While inviting broad membership of a learning group appears desirable and the benefits of drawing together expertise from many disciplines are numerous, it must be remembered that not all groups function cohesively. When considering the composition of a learning group, the aims of the educational activity should be considered, as not all professionals in a palliative care setting will benefit from every activity. Do the professionals have differing, but complementary contributions to make? What is the nature of their professional interaction in the clinical setting? Can a common level of clarity or complexity be found which will suit the learning needs of all members?

Learners should feel comfortable in the group setting, or at least able to participate with a view to becoming more familiar with this type of activity. They should be prepared to work together and helped not to feel in any way threatened (Bliss *et al.* 2000), and they must also be prepared to value the contributions that can be made by all team members. This approach acknowledges the non-hierarchical nature of the interdisciplinary group. Closely knit teams can be resistant to outsiders (Corner 2003) as there may be some tension over roles and responsibilities, but successful interdisciplinary learning relies on participants recognizing the need for and benefit of professional values and cultures being shared. It has been common for any team that has medical specialists within its membership to be driven by these members, with them taking lead roles and dominating the activity. Indeed, Corner (2003) noted when writing about the multidisciplinary team 'while doctors saw themselves in a facilitative role in relation to their ... nurse colleagues, this was from a position of implied seniority'. However, it has also been noted that interdisciplinary teams develop through time and when team dynamics are permitted to evolve (Farrell *et al.* 2001; Corner 2003). This develops a more collaborative and consensual style (Farrell *et al.* 2001), and the dominance seen initially in individual team members can lessen. Continued attention to the group process can help prevent problems arising with group dynamics and can contribute to a successful learning experience.

In clinical specialties, language can be a barrier to effective communication and learning. The group must be able to share a common language, and this can influence its makeup. The subject matter of the training activity will inform the use of language in most instances. Biomedical topics will require a grasp of basic, or more advanced medical terminology, while psycho-social aspects of palliative care can often be taught and discussed by team members with less need for specific technical language. There should be a common understanding of non-technical terms to avoid assumptions being made. This is not to say that team members must be confined by the type of training activity in which they are able to participate; however, as a dynamic, supportive team they should be able to adjust the language employed to achieve inclusivity in the greater proportion of their educational activities.

Attention should also be paid to cultural factors that may arise within the educational setting, whether these are based on ethnicity or organizational influences. In the inclusive world of palliative care, no negative influences should appear due to a group member's sex, age or cultural background, for example, but, unfortunately, this is a problem that may have to be recognized, acknowledged and solved from time to time. The main source of cultural conflict, however, may arise in the form of hierarchical expectations of some group members. While the general trend in health care in the UK is towards an egalitarian interdisciplinary approach to care, elsewhere there may still be a medical-allied health professional–nursing 'pecking order' that can potentially interfere with effective communication and learning in an interdisciplinary education group. Medical staff can attempt to dominate sessions, while nursing staff may feel obliged to defer to their physician colleagues. This is reflected in the often differing contributions of, for example, nurses when in interdisciplinary groups compared with when in nursing subgroups. The contribution of all group members needs to be fostered and any attempts to create a hierarchy of membership within a group actively discouraged.

Within health care, many methods have been employed to facilitate learning, including lectures, case reviews, audit, experiential learning, computer-based study and teaching at the bedside. The subject matter of the activity, as well as the size of group and resources available, often determines the manner in which knowledge and skills are acquired. This variety of educational methods, which can be daunting to those new to planning education sessions, should be viewed positively, as it allows programmes to be tailored to the topic, the clinical setting and the participants in any situation. There has been a shift away from more 'traditional' instructional methods such as the lecture in recent years, with emphasis now being placed on making sessions more active and learner centred. New approaches in teaching methodology have become available—role-play, small group discussion, video-based case studies and computer-assisted learning are just a few examples. The rise in popularity of problem-based learning has also proved to be a convenient and efficient way of involving the learner more in their own education. All forms of curriculum delivery are equally valid and useful, providing they are used appropriately, and all can be used in the interdisciplinary team setting.

Equally important, however, is training of the individuals facilitating a learning activity. It is no longer acceptable to believe the dreadful old medical axiom of 'see one, do one, teach one', and the fact that one may have considerable clinical experience and factual knowledge about a subject does not necessarily lead to one being an effective teacher. This has been recognized and there is now strong support for the 'training the trainers' approach to education. In addition, with the increase in popularity of reflective practice, educators are now being involved in 360° feedback programmes, where they receive anonymous, honest comments on aspects of their practice from a range of individuals with whom they come into contact at work. This can be challenging to the educator, but serves to facilitate the reflective process and identify areas for consideration, change or further training (see Fig. 10.1).

One important adjunct to successful interdisciplinary learning is reflective practice, a concept that has been discussed within education circles since the first half of the last century and which has become very much more popular over the past decade. Reflection involves approaching a situation or problem in a particular manner. It relates to a complex and deliberate process of thinking about and interpreting experience, either demanding or rewarding, in order to learn from it (Atkins and Murphy 1995). It has been said that members of professions develop by reflecting on their practice (Schon 1983), i.e. thinking specifically about what we do and how we do it, and combining this with our related knowledge and experience. However, 'reflective practice is more than just thoughtful practice, it is the process of turning thoughtful practice into a potential learning situation' (Jarvis 1992). This method of learning can be used by the team either to look at situations already encountered or in preparation for those anticipated in order that good standards can be enhanced and the team develops in their role of providing excellent patient care. Reflection can be challenging—many professionals can perceive it as being threatening or critical of their practice—but should be rewarding both clinically and professionally if it is approached in a supportive, non-judgemental atmosphere with the primary goal being that of learning.

Finally, another concept which has been discussed in the literature is that of the 'player manager' (Wilson and Pirrie 2000), a committed individual in the

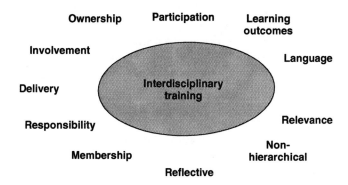

**Fig. 10.1** The facets of interdisciplinary training.

team who, as a 'hands-on' clinician often with a considerable amount of professional and personal experience, helps to create an environment open to learning being part of usual practice. Seeing a skilled and competent professional in the clinical setting can raise enthusiasm and encourage other members of staff to ask questions. This less structured form of team learning can be equally valuable in helping both individuals and the team develop in their professional roles within the organization.

## User involvement in training

For centuries, clinicians have realized that their patients can teach them a great deal. Every patient encountered in clinical practice has something to teach the practitioner, but it is the responsibility of the professional to take heed of what they are being taught. Palliative medicine in particular lends itself to the participation of patients and their carers in some aspects of ongoing education (see Chapter 4 of this volume).

The experience of a life-threatening illness cannot be communicated to professionals through a lecture or PC-based self-directed learning, although theoretical teaching is still more common in palliative care in the undergraduate setting due to a shortage of both suitably skilled staff and clinical attachments to facilitate such teaching (Lloyd-Williams and Field 2002; Lloyd-Williams and Carter 2003; Lloyd-Williams and Macleod 2004); however, through patient narrative and group discussion, the nuances of being 'a palliative care patient' can be identified and explored. Case studies and video interviews can be useful tools to highlight recurrent themes and commonly experienced problems to professionals. With thought and planning, at suitable times with appropriate participants, users can be a valuable resource to the interdisciplinary team developing their practice. Such methods are already being employed in the undergraduate setting (Wee *et al.* 2001) where palliative care lends itself well to integrated teaching covering communication skills, reflective practice and medical ethics (Field and Wee 2002), but could equally be used in postgraduate interdisciplinary learning.

Involving patients and carers in training sessions within palliative care can, however, be problematic. Professionals worry that many patients are ill with advanced disease and have a limited survival, that they may not be physically well enough to participate in education programmes or that, due to the emotional burdens associated with incurable illness, even considering user involvement in teaching and education is in some way unethical. However, users often welcome the opportunity to share their experiences with health professionals. Certainly, patients may gain from the knowledge that their participation may benefit patients in the future. They are given the opportunity to 'have their say' about many issues and to comment on both the process and delivery of care from the viewpoint of the recipient. Such information can be incredibly valuable to the team in evaluating, reflecting upon and adapting both the type of care they provide and the manner in which it is delivered.

## Effects of interdisciplinary training on team dynamics

A move towards more interdisciplinary training within a team is a logical progression of education strategy given current understanding. Consideration should be given, however, to how such a change may impact on the team and the manner in which it functions. Such an approach can be beneficial, by increasing a sense of ownership on professional development as already mentioned, but also as a forum for problem solving within the team and to share the burden of work—both clinical and educational. The aim is that, through interdisciplinary learning, team building occurs which, in turn, should lead to a more effective team.

It needs to be recognized that interdisciplinary training can be perceived as threatening by some as it seeks to blur professional boundaries. It can, however, empower team members to trust and be more tolerant of others and encourage willingness to share responsibility (Nolan 1995). The aim is not to 'change the roles of the team but to acknowledge and negotiate them' (Stiefel 2003), but it must be accepted that not all teams function effectively, and not all team members have perfect relationships with all their colleagues. There may be individual groups with a 'particular disciplinary axe to grind' (Wilson and Pirrie 2000). Such hidden dynamics can be destructive to the group process and can adversely affect the progress of the team in its educational endeavours. It has been said that, in some areas of medicine, 'dying people are not the real problem', emphasizing that the dynamics of the workplace play a major role in a practitioner's sense of well-being (Vachon 1987). It should be stressed, however, that an interdisciplinary approach to both training and team working should not be assumed to be a remedy for existing tensions within a team, though an understanding of team dynamics can help. In fact, it might be appropriate to develop an interdisciplinary focus on team dynamics as part of any training programme.

## Conclusion

Palliative medicine has developed based on the axis of keeping the patient central and the existence of an interdisciplinary team core which positively impacts on the provision of quality care. For many years, professions have been taught, and have subsequently developed, in isolation, which has often resulted in misunderstanding, misconception and, in some instances, mistrust. To achieve truly effective professional partnerships with colleagues and, in turn, to provide coordinated, quality palliative care, a move towards inter-disciplinary training in teams is not only desired, but essential.

# References

Atkins S and Murphy K (1995). Reflective practice. *Nursing Standard* **9** (45), 31–35.

Barr H and Waterton S (1996). *Interprofessional Education in Health and Social Care in the United Kingdom: Report of a CAIPE Survey.* Centre for the Advancement of Interprofessional Education, London.

Beard RM and Hartley J (1984). *Teaching and Learning in Higher Education.* Paul Chapman, London.

Bliss J, Cowley S and While A (2000). Interprofessional working in palliative care in the community: a review of the literature. *Journal of Interprofessional Care* **14**, 281–290.

Carpenter J (1995). Interprofessional education for medical and nursing students: evaluation of a programme. *Medical Education* **29**, 265–72.

Clark PG (1993). A typology of multidisciplinary education in gerontology and geriatrics: are we really doing what we say we are? *Journal of Interprofessional Care* **7**, 217–227.

Corner J (2003). The multidisciplinary team—fact or fiction? *European Journal of Palliative Care* **10**, S10–s12.

Crawford GB and Price SD (2003). Team working: palliative care as a model of interdisciplinary practice. *Medical Journal of Australia* **179**, S32–S34.

Department of Health (2000). *A Health Service of All the Talents: Developing the NHS Workforce.* Department of Health, London.

Department of Health (2001). *Investment and Reform for NHS Staff: Taking Forward the NHS Plan.* Department of Health, London.

Farrell MP, Schmitt MH and Heinemann GD (2001). Informal roles and the stages of interdisciplinary team development. *Journal of Interprofessional Care* **15**, 281–295.

Field D and Wee B (2002). Preparation for palliative care: teaching about death, dying and bereavement in UK medical schools 2000–2001. *Medical Education* **36**, 561–567.

Horsburgh M, Lamdin R and Williamson E (2001). Multiprofessional learning: the attitudes of medical, nursing and pharmacy students to shared learning. *Medical Education* **35**, 876–83.

Jarvis P (1992). Reflective practice and nursing. *Nursing Education Today* **12**, 174–181.

Knowles M (1973). *The Adult Learner—A Neglected Species.* Gulf Publishing, Houston, TX.

Lloyd-Williams M and Carter YH (2003). General practice vocational training in the UK: what teaching is given in palliative care? *Palliative Medicine* **17**, 616–620.

Lloyd-Williams M and Field D (2002). Are undergraduate nurses taught palliative care during their training? *Nurse Education Today* **22**, 589–592.

Lloyd-Williams M and Macleod RD (2004). A systematic review of teaching and learning in palliative care within the undergraduate curriculum. *Medical Teacher* **26**, 683–690.

McMichael P and Gilloran A (1984). *Exchanging Views: Courses in Collaboration.* Moray House College, Edinburgh.

Nolan M (1995). Towards an ethos of interdisciplinary practice. *British Medical Journal* **312**, 305–306.

Parker GM (1994). *Cross-functional Teams: Working With Allies, Enemies and Other Strangers*. Jossey-Bass Publishers, San Francisco, pp. 31–40.

Parsell G and Bligh J (1999). The development of a questionnaire to assess the readiness of health care students for interprofessional learning (RIPLS). *Medical Education* **33**, 95–100.

Richmond D (1988). Preparing students for continuing education. In: Cox KR and Ewan CE, ed. *The Medical Teacher*. Churchill Livingstone, New York, p. 136.

Schon DA (1983). *The Reflective Practitioner*. Basic Books, New York.

Stiefel F (2003). Response: the multidisciplinary team—fact or fiction? *European Journal of Palliative Care* 10, S12–s13.

Vachon M (1987). *Occupational Stress in the Care of the Critically Ill*. Hemisphere Publishing Company, New York, pp. 51–73.

Wee B, Hillier R, Coles C, Mountford B, Sheldon F and Turner P (2001). Palliative care: a suitable setting for undergraduate interprofessional education. *Palliative Medicine* **15**, 487–492.

Wilson V and Pirrie A (2000). *Multidisciplinary Teamworking: Beyond the Barriers? A Review of the Issues*. Scottish Council for Research in Education, Glasgow.

# 11

# Ethical issues in multidisciplinary teamwork within palliative care

*Bobbie Farsides*

One could claim that palliative care practitioners are to be congratulated for having a fairly sophisticated approach to the ethical issues involved in patient care. The literature of palliative care ethics is well developed compared with some other health care specialties, and practitioners and academics in the field have contributed to the broader ethical debates relating to death and dying. In Britain, both the Association of Palliative Medicine and The National Council for Palliative Care have active ethics committees that regularly survey the issues that arise in the field.

However, when considering the working of multidisciplinary teams, it is important to appreciate that there may be ethical issues that arise which are specific to the very issue of team working that have received less attention. This problem is not unique to palliative care. In many morally contested areas of health care, we have been slow to take adequate account of the moral views and experiences of practitioners operating within teams.

For this reason, this chapter will not offer a survey of the everyday ethical issues facing palliative care teams. Nor will it provide an exhaustive account of *how* teams deal with such problems. Rather it will look closely at the challenges individuals might have to face when they attempt to work together in what can be a highly morally charged environment. Thus the focus will be on the implications for individuals of working as part of a team, moreover as part of a team that will almost inevitably confront moral or ethical issues in their work.

Other chapters in this volume have explored the nature and composition of the multidisciplinary team, and have given substance to this readily employed label. Whilst it is important for an ethicist to have a realistic and accurate understanding of the nature of such a team in terms of the professional groups represented, the hierarchies and separations of power present, and the nature of the practical tasks taken on, the starting point for the ethicist is that a team is a group of individuals with each individual a moral agent in their own right. As such, the individual practitioner will have beliefs, views, ideas and projects which in a substantial way track what they think about the world and how they categorize actions and events as right or wrong, morally acceptable or unacceptable, forbidden or allowed. A challenge facing the individual is to reconcile their personal moral views with those required by, or most readily identified with, their professional role and their membership of a larger moral unit—the team.

Similarly, the challenge for the team (and in some cases the team leader) is to ensure that individuals can contribute productively to the activities of the team whilst remaining true to the beliefs and values they hold as individuals. This challenge might become particularly real if the team has a strong philosophy or ethos which particular individuals find hard to accept, or at least wish to challenge. To consider another possibility, if the team decides to change or modify its philosophy in the light of external factors, an individual might feel that their personal philosophy no longer fits as well with that of the team. In this case, the conflict between the values of the team and those of the individual might give rise to a conflict between individual autonomy and group membership/identification.

## Autonomy—the value we cannot ignore

On a number of occasions over the years, I have questioned the pre-eminence of autonomy as a moral value in the northern European context (Farsides 1994, 1998). I have similarly explored the consequences for patients and carers of putting into practice a theoretical regard for respect of patient autonomy (Farsides 1996). On this occasion, however, I am tempted to argue that we need to care *more* about the autonomy of individuals working within palliative care teams than is sometimes evident.

Autonomy is a word that is utilized a great deal in the palliative care world. A basic literature search will reveal numerous articles in which the terms autonomy and palliative care appear side by side, and as such the work in this area reflects a persisting interest in autonomy within health care and bioethics more generally.

It used to be the case that people were happy to define autonomy as something akin to its etymological root of 'self-rule', with a clear emphasis placed on the need to be independent of thought and action if one were to be considered autonomous. However, definitions of autonomy have become more sophisticated over time, with many commentators moving away from a simple correlation between autonomy and substantive independence (e.g. Dworkin 1988). This is helpful in the present context because, if we were to define autonomy as some form of self-governance that relies on the individual remaining sovereign, self-determining and independent of the influence of others, it becomes potentially problematic where one is asking an individual to operate as part of a team. With contemporary definitions, it is possible to reconcile the autonomy of the individual with their loyalty and commitment to the larger group.

Happily the more sophisticated concepts of autonomy take realistic account of our associations with others. They also acknowledge that we construct our moral lives in such a way as to preclude the possibility of always acting independently. Interdependence and interconnection are seen as a reality and not necessarily a problem. Furthermore, modern accounts of autonomy are capable of accommodating the idea that moral agents make choices to attach themselves to groups and/or projects that then demand that they do not always follow a self-determined path. Values such as loyalty, friendship and fidelity may all require that at times we make choices that we would not make were we functioning purely on the basis of individual interest or concern for personal values.

These ideas contribute to our understanding of how someone might align themselves to a set of beliefs, or identify themselves with a group which has a strong and prescriptive grip over their choices and actions. So, for example, an individual might autonomously choose to define themselves as a member of a religious group which has clear dietary laws and strict rules governing the observance of the Sabbath. Because they value their group membership and accept the teachings of their faith, they do not feel that being governed by the laws of the religion is a threat to their autonomy. Indeed, they may feel that their autonomy is severely under threat if and when others seek to undermine or over-ride their decision to be governed by their religion in certain areas of life.

A religious group comes together because it shares fundamental beliefs or articles of faith. In this case, group membership is in an important sense determined by what the people in the group believe. Within the group, there may be differences in interpretation or ritual, but there needs to be some fundamental basis upon which individuals define themselves as members of that particular religion as opposed to any other. If the fundamental articles of faith are challenged, it might be suggested that those who challenge them have moved outside the religion. Thus there may be limits upon the extent to which an individual is able to act autonomously and still define themselves as a *bona fide* member of this particular group.

## Common purpose

Somewhat differently from members of a religious fraternity, a team is a group of people brought together by a common task, who (unless they are engaged in a pursuit clearly governed by rules) need to negotiate and adopt ways of working towards that task and associated goals. This negotiation might be more straightforward if the members of the team share certain fundamental beliefs but, irrespective of this, their common purpose will be what binds them together.

Whilst the individual might value being a member of a successful team, and wish to promote an ethos of team working, this in itself would not be their primary purpose in their working life. Instead, the team works together to achieve certain goals and promote certain values in pursuit of their purpose. To borrow Kant's terminology, one could say that the team is a means to an end as opposed to an end in itself. In the palliative care setting, one could say that the team exists to provide good palliative care in the interest of those for whom the team cares.

The palliative care team might not be one's only focus of allegiance in one's professional life. It is telling that when asked to define oneself in terms of one's professional persona, it would be more usual to name a constituent part of the team than to refer simply to being a team member, e.g. a nurse working in a hospital palliative care team, a social worker operating within a hospice-based team. In these cases, it begins to sound as if the individual describes themselves as being part of a team within a team. This is of course a possible feature of any group that defines itself as multi- or cross-disciplinary. The important point to bear in mind, however, is that the teams represented within the teams may share different values and have different perspectives on how to interpret and achieve their shared goals

## Common beliefs

A palliative care team in common with other teams operating within a health care setting is a group of people with different forms of expertise and different professional affiliations coming together to pursue a common purpose in the interests of a shared client group. However, it might be the case that group membership in a palliative care setting has commonly been assumed to denote more than this. Unlike many other areas of health care, we speak quite freely of the 'palliative care philosophy' or the 'palliative care movement'. Furthermore, most practitioners could give a good account of what the philosophy entails in terms of beliefs about what one ought and ought not to do as a palliative care practitioner, with the 'ought' in this sentence covering moral as well as practical considerations.

One could argue that this is an unusual feature of this particular area of health care. Beyond very broad generalities, one would not attempt to attribute a commonality of views to colleagues working together in orthopaedics or dentistry, for example, and in other areas such as childbirth or psychiatry the differences between practitioners have been more interesting than the similarities. Yet the view persists in many quarters that palliative care practitioners think as one over a significant and important range of issues.

One could offer a variety of tentative explanations for this apparent difference. Some point to the religious roots of the modern hospice movement and the remaining influence of faith-based foundations to suggest that the notion of shared belief outlined above transfers across in to the caring context. One could point to the influence of particular pioneers, who in fighting against a medical establishment disinclined to hear their message developed sophisticated holistic defences of the need for this particular form of medical intervention. One might hypothesize about the way in which hospices in the past remained largely outside of and separate from the larger health care system, thus allowing a certain degree of insularity to prevail.

Others have addressed the history of the movement in a way that is beyond the scope of this chapter (see www.hospice-history.org.uk); the interesting thing is that there is perceived to be a *movement* to study. Be it real or assumed, it is a commonly held view that being a palliative care practitioner is about more than sharing a common goal; it could also entail sharing some fundamental beliefs about what is and is not permissible in the pursuit of those goals. The interesting questions that then arise are whether this common view (real or not) is compatible with other prevailing views in our society, and to what extent an individual who does not share what is assumed to be the commonly held views can work successfully within the team.

## Working together

In the context of multidisciplinary team working, we could argue that *if* there is independent evidence to suggest that the goals of the team are valuable, and that they can be best secured by working as a team, each individual has a good (professional) reason to participate as a team member. Having participated in an appropriate decision-making process, the individual should then move in the direction the team feels is appropriate. To translate this into palliative care terms, if the good of patients and families can best be secured by working as a team, the individual has a good (professional) reason to participate as a team member, and to carry out the tasks that contribute to the goals that the team is pursuing.

One could further argue that one of the keys to being a good team member is to be a 'team player', i.e. someone who is prepared to accept and play by the rules of the game in the interests of the team doing well. The interesting question then becomes one regarding the extent to which the rules of the game require an individual to prioritize the beliefs and values promoted by the group over and above their own, if and when the two conflict; or, in situations where responsibility ultimately lies with one individual, the extent to which others are prepared to accept that this individual's views will prevail even when their views are very different from one's own.

## The common goal

The definition of palliative care offered by the World Health Organization (2004) and the familiar phraseology of pioneers such as the late Dame Cicely Saunders (Saunders 1996) inform us that palliative care is the holistic care of patients and their families once the patient's illness is no longer open to cure. The goal of treatment is to alleviate or at least control symptoms, offer pain relief and cater to the psycho-social, spiritual and emotional needs of the service users, be they patient or family, in the interests of enabling the patient to live with their terminal diagnosis and the family to survive the death.

Even put this simply, one can see that there might be room for disagreement within the team about such things as which problems to treat as priorities, which of two incommensurate goals to pursue, who to prioritize when two potential clients' needs are at odds, or how best to construct a service to deliver these goods. This is in a sense the stuff of everyday work, and the experienced team will have learnt how and when to remould itself, maybe on a daily basis, so that different members become key players at different times and in relation to different problems and issues. In a sense, the disagreements that occur will be professional disagreements resulting from practitioners having different views about what is most important at any one stage and how to deal with it. Such disagreements will be played out against a background of shared values and goals that ensure that each individual and subgroup remains committed to the ultimate goal of providing care, alleviating suffering and enriching life.

However, there are some differences of opinion that are not essentially professional but are instead profoundly moral, and here the impact upon the team and the skills required to deal with or accommodate them may be quite different. This fact is bought into sharp relief when one ponders the obvious fact that as well as making the remaining life of the patient as good as possible, the palliative care team will also be involved with the death of the patient. As such, the team will be involved in caring for a patient at a time in their life when his/her own spiritual and moral beliefs may come to the fore. Furthermore, the carer may have specific moral and/or religious beliefs about how (if at all) the death of any one individual, or death more generally, should be managed. Whilst an individual practitioner's views have always been relevant to how they contribute to discussions and decisions relating to patient care, it is now important that practitioners understand that their different moral views might come to be played out during a time of radical change.

If the law is changed to allow either physician-assisted suicide or voluntary euthanasia, palliative care practitioners will be faced with a range of difficult moral decisions as individuals, as team members and as members of larger organizations. Such a change would be a huge challenge for a team to face, but one cannot afford to be complacent about the challenges that a process exploring the possibility of change might also pose.

## Exploring the commonality of belief

It is probably accurate to state that the palliative care philosophy as broadly perceived has set itself against the idea of medical intervention in assisted dying. Having said this, I have heard experienced practitioners complain at the adoption of the term 'assisted dying' by those advocating assisted suicide and euthanasia. Their point is that palliative care assists people to die well, but it does so without killing them.

Even in the most recent stage of the public debate on Lord Joffe's proposed bill, many of those most publicly and forcibly objecting to the proposed changes came from a palliative care background[1]. However, recent research has also indicated that within the movement there is a broader spread of views than might be suggested by some of those who speak on behalf of their fellow professionals (Shale 2005).

This is not the occasion on which to explore the ethical fundamentals of this issue further. However, the possibility of disagreement within the group on this important issue, coupled with pre-conceptions about the group's views that may or may not be accurate, provides an interesting context within which to discuss the moral complexities of team work.

In other contexts, I have carried out empirical research which suggests that even within teams with a publicly recognized ethos and highly successful working relationship, there is room for tension regarding ethically charged issues. This tension may be either personally experienced, or if it becomes more problematic can have implications for the working life of the team. If a team characterizes itself in terms of a shared moral perspective on matters of importance to their work, it can be problematic for the individual involved and the team when someone 'steps out of line'. If on the other hand the team is cohesive in its moral view but at odds with the larger organization within which it exists, the team may be characterized as 'problematic' and its position may be undermined.

## Personal views in a professional context

An individual's moral views are not always predictable, nor are they always obvious or accessible to those with whom they work. I have been privileged over many years to hear a wide variety of health care professionals and bio-medical scientists speak openly and in some detail about how they feel about the ethical issues that are raised by their work[2]. In the course of these conversations, interviews and group discussion sessions, I have heard colleagues propound views that others consider incompatible with the work they do. I have heard individuals who work in teams that are considered to be cutting edge and ethically adventurous admit to serious moral reservations and demonstrate a moral conservatism in terms of their own views and actions (Williams *et al.* 2002*a*). I have met colleagues who when speaking in a group context toe the party line when I know that in their private interviews their views are clearly at odds with one another and the 'group speak' they seem to feel obliged to express. I have personally been criticized for suggesting that there are no logical barriers to people in certain contexts thinking in ways that are seen as unusual and maybe unacceptable (Randall 1999). As a result of all of this, I have come to believe that the most successful teams are those which accommodate a broad range of views on important topics, but this variety can be hard to manage organizationally, and it can exact a heavy cost on individual members of the team and on the leadership (Williams *et al.* 2002*b*).

This is not to say that all views can or should be tolerated within a team. There is a sense in which views that militate against successfully working towards the team's defined goals, or which undermine the fundamental values upon which a team's vision is based, cannot be compatible with continued membership of the group. Defining the exact content of such views is a subtle and complicated exercise, and one needs to avoid assumptions about what people need to believe in order to do X or Y, but a successful team will be able to establish which of its fundamental values are non-negotiable.

## Expressing oneself

In moral philosophy, it is interesting to explore the difference between holding a view, expressing a view and acting upon that view. In a liberal democratic society, a significant component of individual liberty is the right to hold whatever views we see fit, and in many cases we have the right to act on those views even if others consider them completely irrational, mistaken or maybe even dangerous. Thus in English law, a competent individual can refuse medical treatment for reasons that others consider unfathomable, even if the consequences of doing so are predicted to be dire. The law intervenes only when our competence is in question or when our choice of action or the views we express entail a harm to others. In line with John Stuart Mill's thinking as set out in *On Liberty* (1859), we are prepared to allow that some matters are properly understood as *private* and as such should not be subject to the interference of others until and unless they are accompanied by a significant harm to those same or different others. However, it is not always easy to separate the private from the public, and for health care professionals working in morally charged environments there might sometimes be a complex relationship between what they believe as a private individual and what is required of them as a professional.

## Thinking outside the box

Consider the scenario, outlined in Box 11.1. The issue here is not whether Philip is right or wrong in terms of his views, but rather whether he was right to express those views in the way that he has, given his responsibilities within the team that he essentially leads. As one is often reminded, responsibility is the flip side of autonomy. Whilst one is free to hold ones own views irrespective of the views of the team, one has to acknowledge that the expression of those views may impact upon the team, and one needs to take responsibility for judging the implications of this fact.

In this case, it is certainly unfortunate that this is the first time Philip has aired his views on this sensitive subject, and he has done so publicly and apparently without consultation. Colleagues might regret or even resent the fact that Philip had never shared his views with them. Alternatively, even if they do not feel personally affronted that they did not know where he stood, they may consider he has wronged them by speaking in his role of Chief

---

**Box 11.1 SPEAKING OUT OF LINE**

Philip has recently been appointed Chief Executive of a well-established hospice in a small northern town. His background is in social work, initially in care of the elderly but in recent years in palliative care. He is a larger than life character who has galvanized the staff, and has done a great deal to reawaken the local community's interest in fundraising for the hospice.

Last week, Philip gave an interview to a local journalist who, having finished asking him about the new day care centre, asked him what he thought of the recent attempts to introduce some measure of assisted dying into English law. Initially Philip presented the 'party line', stating that good palliative care could remove the desire to end ones life prematurely, therefore the government should be spending its time on funding palliative care, not passing bills to legalize assisted suicide. However, when pressed by the journalist, he agreed that he could see a place for physician-assisted suicide in a small number of cases, and he could anticipate a point in the future when his hospice would care for patients who requested such help. On Saturday morning, the local paper reported that 'local hospice could offer to help patients end their lives'.

Returning to work after the weekend, Philip is met by a storm of protest from senior colleagues, and in the staff canteen he does not meet with his usual enthusiastic welcome. However, he also receives a number of supportive E-mails, and one of the patients congratulates him on having said what he thinks.

Executive on a matter they consider to be unexplored within their organization. If this is the case, one has to wonder how someone of his experience has placed himself in this position. However, one also needs to ask whether there are specific reasons particular to the nature of the topic that help explain how this situation could have arisen.

It might be that the taboo nature of the topic of assisted dying means that it is rarely if ever raised within a working environment such as the hospice Philip is associated with. This may be regrettable given the public debate that is brewing but, given the very real day-to-day issues Philip has to deal with, it may not have been one of his priorities to canvas staff views on the issue or share his own. Having said that, it might rather be the case that Philip has felt it unwise to share his views, sensing them to be at odds with those of important people he needs to work alongside in his new role. To put it more strongly, Philip may have been wary of compromising his position by taking what he assumes to be an unpopular stance on an issue that has previously not been central to the current agenda.

Whatever the reasons, one could claim that a mistake has been made. An individual whose views could (albeit mistakenly) be taken to be representative of the organization they manage has made a public statement that is based on his own moral and professional judgement. However, would Philip have met the same response if he had said that he could never see a day when hospices would be involved in assisted dying, or that he saw no need to legalize such interventions irrespective of the role of hospices? Would such a story have made the headlines?

I would suggest that such a statement would have been seen as much less newsworthy by the local journalist, but this is by the by. More importantly, I would also suggest that Philip would have met a rather different reaction from the majority of his colleagues in the wake of such a statement. It is uncontroversial to present what is taken to be the orthodox view, even if there are growing numbers of dissenters. Yet, he would still have been making a public statement based upon his own moral and professional judgement. The difference is that it is now more in step with the institutional or group view as commonly perceived. Whilst some colleagues might quietly hold to a different view, what he would have said in this case would have allowed many of his team to remain within their comfort zone. This does not make the issue unproblematic, it just has fewer direct ramifications for the team.

What a case such as this demonstrates is the need to confront the issue of how to accommodate a range of views within an organization, and how to allow individuals to express those views whilst still being part of the team pursuing the goals they hold in common. It is also important to recognize that subjects upon which people have chosen not to focus in the past might, through changes in circumstance, become fairly urgent topics for consideration. Thus, in the case of assisted dying, the time may have come when it becomes wise to have the range of 'what if . . . ' conversations that have seemed unnecessary and maybe even inadvisable in the past. However, one should not underestimate how difficult this may be to manage as a process, and one needs to be clear about what one hopes to achieve. Essentially, the process should be directed towards enabling the team to confront, explore and hopefully absorb differences in moral attitude towards an issue that will possibly become of direct practical concern in the relatively near future. This is a limited goal in the first instance, but this is surely appropriate given the importance of the issue and the range of beliefs and attitudes that may realistically exist within any one team.

So, one could argue that a first step towards ensuring that a team survives and indeed thrives in a time of moral and or legal uncertainty or change is to break any silence that has previously existed around the subject in question. Organizations need to give their teams permission and create space to discuss morally challenging issues in a context where people feel safe and free to express and explore a variety of views (Alderson *et al.* 2002). If it is known to be the case that a particular view is held by the majority of members of a particular team, this is not in itself evidence that this view is 'right', and it is still necessary to give voice to opposing positions. If there is a minority holding dissenting views, their ideas need to be aired, but this must be done without making the individuals in this significant subgroup feel vulnerable. In some situations, a trained ethicist or external facilitator might be needed to give voice to views that have not traditionally been aired in the palliative care setting.

## Speaking out of line

Whilst no one can condemn Philip for his views, or for his predictions for the future, one must understand that there are good reasons for him not to express his personal views when speaking in his professional capacity. *Within* the organization he may have a responsibility to use his position to prompt discussion of a sensitive issue. He may have an important role in making others feel free to express various views that differ from the received wisdom. However, given the range of issues for which he remains responsible, and the importance of having a good relationship with his staff, he should if necessary step back and leave the job of facilitating a process of sharing and exploring moral issues to disinterested experts.

However, it is possible that Philip's role could become important again further down the line. If the law were to change, and it became permissible for doctors to assist in the suicide of their patients, individual health care professionals and the organizations within which they worked would have important decisions to make. In the case of the movement as a whole, palliative care practitioners would need to decide what role, if any, they were willing to take in the process of assisted suicide, and on the basis of that decision individual institutions, teams and practitioners would have to decide where they stood. However, at this stage where the issue remains one of forming and sharing views, there is good reason for any one team to concentrate upon hearing and listening to the views of its members rather than publicizing those views abroad, even in terms of contributing to a national debate.

I make this final point knowing that it will provoke a reaction from some of those who have taken time and trouble to contribute well thought out and articulate responses to the debate around assisted dying. I am not suggesting that it is in any sense wrong for them to do so, nor would I wish a debate to proceed without the expertise of palliative care practitioners being given its due weight, rather my point is that a robust defence of the *views* or *beliefs* of the groups should never be allowed to impede the achievement of the *goals* of the group, or the task of the team.

To illustrate this point, I can return to my earlier claim that it would not be unproblematic if Philip had vehemently opposed the idea that assisted suicide should be legalized and stated that it would never occur in 'his' hospice, even if this would have meant he earned the agreement of most of his staff. The problem would then be with the image the institution presented to future patients and their families, some of whom would welcome such a change and possibly consider availing of such a service. A clear and persistent moral objection by a local service provider might well translate in peoples' minds to the idea that in future they would have to make a choice between assisted dying or palliative care and, as colleagues in The Netherlands have demonstrated, this need not be the case given the willingness to provide euthanasia within some Dutch nursing home palliative care units.

If as has been suggested by the recent House of Lord's committee the ultimate decision on this issue is one for society as a whole, groups of health care professionals within this society must ensure that in exercising their right to enter the debate, they do not jeopardize their ability to welcome into their care all those who would benefit from it, irrespective of how their views might differ. It is therefore a challenge facing multidisciplinary teams to encourage freedom of speech without repercussion *within* the team and temper freedom of speech in the public arena in order to remain effective in their primary role as providers of care to all comers within their community. However, as previously mentioned, there is a morally relevant distinction between holding a view, expressing a view and acting upon a view, and it is now necessary to consider this final component.

## Walking the talk

Assume for the sake of argument that the law was going to change to allow carefully regulated physician-assisted suicide. For the purposes of discussion, the exact proposals are unimportant, and one need not form a personal view on whether or not this was a good thing in order to consider the implications for any particular team of palliative care practitioners. What we will assume for the sake of argument is that the preceding public debate was conducted fairly and transparently, that parliament approached the issue with due seriousness and that the result was unambiguous. What we have, therefore, is a democratically mandated change in the law giving people a right to demand an intervention within a health care setting which many will continue to believe either morally wrong or at least ill advised. As such, this does not differ dramatically from the case relating to the provision of termination of pregnancy.

The question then arises of what could and should be demanded of individual practitioners and teams given that legalisation will not take the moral heat out of the subject of assisted dying. Many practitioners will remain opposed in principle to the change; others will fear the societal and professional impact of such a change.

In very broad terms, the issue is addressed through giving practitioners a legal right to object conscientiously to participating in procedures to which they are morally opposed; but even this is not as straightforward as it seems. It is not necessarily the case that an individual and the team within which they work will share a definition of what counts as 'participation'. Has a nurse participated in a termination if she collects drugs from the hospital pharmacy along with the rest of the supplies, or has a nurse participated in physician-assisted suicide if she checks the physician's measurement of the lethal dose when checking all the other drugs? In the course of our research, we have met practitioners who can justify quite significant involvement in processes to which they are morally opposed and those who have gone so far as to leave a discipline in order to avoid involvement in the moral choices the law permits their patients. Neither approach is morally inconsistent, and it is up to the individual and the teams within which they operate to negotiate how this might occur.

I have suggested elsewhere that when it comes to acting upon our moral views in a professional context, we can take one of three approaches—we can be an absolutist, a tolerator or a facilitator (Farsides *et al.* 2004). These categories were derived from empirical data collected as a result of discussing the ethical issues of their work with a range of health care professionals working in what we defined as 'morally contested fields'.

In practice, *absolutists* were rare amongst the groups we studied. These are the people who on the basis of their moral beliefs feel not only that they wish to dissociate themselves from a practice, but also that the practice should not be made available even if it is legally permissible. Their views can be contrasted with those of *tolerators* who may share a basic moral belief that something is wrong, but because that thing is legally permissible and because they respect the autonomy of others who choose options of which they disapprove they 'allow it to happen'. Each of these groups can in turn be contrasted with *facilitators* who do not simply 'allow things to happen' in the sense of not attempting to change the law or not trying to change the provision of care within their institution. Indeed, the facilitator will accompany and assist the autonomous patient in a procedure or course of events the outcome of which is morally objectionable to them.

Thus the views of practitioners range across those who wish to 'keep their own hands clean' and/or shape the world in their own moral image, to those who will prioritize the moral views of another over their own, often at considerable personal cost.

The challenge for the team in the face of this interesting range of views is to incorporate the individuals holding them within the team and to support each of them as far as this is consistent with continuing to pursue the goals the team is designed to achieve, i.e. the provision of health care services to their client group. If the absolutist refuses to partake in the core duties of the team, then their position may be untenable. If they feel unable to give due respect to patients whose choices offend their moral beliefs, their role in the team will need to be addressed. If their public campaigning activities conflict with their professional life, then they and the team may face some difficult decisions. Thus the role of the absolutist and their place within a team that has embraced a tolerant or facilitative approach can be problematic, and our empirical data suggest that many choose to opt out of the fields in which they believe their fundamental moral beliefs will be incompatible with the work they will be required to do. This raises very interesting issues with respect to the group of individuals within palliative care who may choose to take an absolutist moral view towards the deliberate ending of human life.

For the sake of argument, let us assume that absolutists are well represented in Philips's hospice. They have participated vocally in the public debate preceding legalisation, and post-legalisation they have availed of their individual right to object conscientiously to involvement in what they see as medicalized killing. Now, however, they face the possibility of the team of which they are a part deciding to offer this service within their institution. This decision could be reached because of the influence of *tolerators* and *facilitators* within the team who believe that if something is legally permissible it should be available as an option for competent patients who request it. Such a decision would make the team an uncomfortable place for the absolutist to remain, and one can understand why the absolutists might want to work hard to keep the hospice a physician-assisted suicide-free zone. However, if the team ultimately decides to offer physician-assisted suicide, the absolutist has to decide what to do next.

I would like to argue that far from leaving the scene of the proposed moral crime, there might be a moral imperative upon them to remain within the team subject to a real and robust assurance that they will be allowed to protect themselves from direct involvement in procedures to which they have a fundamental moral objection.

This is a lot to ask of the individual, and one could argue that you are inviting them to become *tolerators* as opposed to *absolutists*. There is a certain amount of truth to this claim, although one could allow that the absolutist would continue in their private life to try and change the world such that there was less likelihood of the moral wrong they object to existing. Why then ask for this sacrifice; is it simply to allow that more autonomous individuals get access to good palliative care practitioners whatever the moral views on either side? This is part of but not the whole reason for wanting the absolutist to stay within the team.

I would argue that one of the great advantages of the multidisciplinary team is that each subgroup within it acts as a corrective to the view that any one group of professionals can do everything that is needed for a patient and their family. This corrective mechanism can also work at a moral level. If a range of moral opinions are represented within the team, no one perspective is allowed to prevail to the extent that moral debate and self-examination are replaced by complacency and lack of self-criticism or awareness.

If there is ever to be physician-assisted suicide within the walls of a hospice, I would be grateful for the continued presence of those who find it morally unacceptable and/or socially worrying. Any move away from a traditional moral prohibition would surely feel safer if the views of enthusiasts were tempered by those of tolerators, sceptics and opponents. If this is a valid position to hold, I would advise Philip ahead of any change in the law to find out who exists within his team in terms of their views on the role of hospices in a society that allows physician-assisted suicide, and their personal positions as prospective *absolutists, tolerators and facilitators*. He should then ensure that they remain within his organization for as long as they feel that they can combine their individual moral views with the shared pursuit of the team's goals. I would also ask him to remind his colleagues that their goal is to care for people whose disease will lead to their death, and the death they choose may not be the death their carers would want for them, but if it is legally permissible and someone is prepared to facilitate it they have that option.

We live in interesting times. As I write this chapter, an execution in the USA has been postponed because no medical practitioner would agree to administer the lethal injection[3]. The power of a strongly held moral objection should not be underestimated, but nor should the political will to achieve that which the law allows. I have suggested that palliative care teams who are opposed to assisted dying should be as cautious in expressing their views as those who support it. Strong expressions on either side of a polarized moral debate potentially alienate parts of the community one exists to serve. However, *within* teams, I urge people to discuss and make obvious the views that exist, partly in order to test the claims to moral uniformity that are so often made. Also, if the law were to change, I ask the biggest commitment of all, that those who remain morally opposed to the change consider remaining within their teams even if the team decides to offer physician-assisted suicide to the very small number of patients who may request it.

## References

Alderson P, Farsides B and Williams C (2002). Examining ethics in practice: health service professionals' evaluation of in-hospital ethics seminars. *Nursing Ethics* 9, 508–520.

Dworkin G (1988). *Theory and Practice of Autonomy.* Cambridge University Press, Cambridge.

Farsides B (1994). Midwifery, autonomy and responsibility. In: Budd S and Sharma U, ed. *The Healing Bond.* Routledge, London, pp. 42–61.

Farsides B (1996). Euthanasia: failure or autonomy? *International Journal of Palliative Nursing* 2 (2), April–June.

Farsides B (1998). Autonomy and its implications for palliative care: a northern European perspective. *Palliative Medicine* 12, 147–151.

Farsides B, Alderson P and Williams C (2004). Aiming towards 'moral' equilibrium: health care professionals' views on working within the morally contested field of antenatal screening. *Journal of Medical Ethics* 30, 505–509.

Randall F (1999). Reply to Farsides' editorial: palliative care—euthanasia-free zone. *Journal of Medical Ethics* 25, 221–223.

Saunders C (1996). Into the valley of the shadow of death: a personal therapeutic journey. *British Medical Journal* 313, 1599–1601.

Shale S (2005). Exploring common ground: alternative views on assistance to die. Emergent issues at symposia for hospice staff. (Unpublished data presented at Help the Hospices Annual Conference, Harrogate, UK.)

Williams C, Alderson P and Farsides B (2002a). Dilemmas encountered by health care practitioners offering nuchal translucency screening: a qualitative case study. *Prenatal Diagnosis* 2, 216–220.

Williams C, Alderson P and Farsides B (2002b). Drawing the line in prenatal screening and testing: health practitioners' discussions. *Health, Risk and Society* 4, 61–75.

World Health Organization (2004). Definition of palliative care at http://www.who.int/cancer/palliative/definition/en/

. [1] hhttp://www.publications.parliament.uk/pa/ld/ldasdy.htm

. [2] These opportunities arose through my work on the following projects: 'Cross currents in genetics and ethics around the millennium' (Wellcome Trust Biomedical Ethics Programme. Grant no. 056009). 'Facilitating choice, framing choice: experiences of staff working in pre-implantation genetic diagnosis'. (Wellcome Trust Biomedical Ethics Programme. Grant no. 074935). 'Mapping stem cell innovation in action: from bench to bedside'.(ESRC grant no. RES340250003).

. [3] I refer to the case of the convicted murderer Michael Morales whose execution was postponed indefinitely in February 2006. It was widely reported that although no medical professional would come forward to administer the lethal drug, the majority of Californians remained supportive of capital punishment.

## 12

# Legal issues of multiprofessional teamwork

*Jonathan Montgomery*

Legal issues may arise in multiprofessional teams in a number of ways. Sometimes there will be particular functions that the law reserves for specific team members. An example would be the use of prescription-only medicines, where the general rule is that only doctors may authorize their use (although provisions exist to extend prescribing powers to members of other health professions in certain circumstances). Here the role of law is to define the roles of different members of the team. This can hinder the development of successful teams by creating hierarchies and demarcations that will not necessarily reflect the most productive dynamics amongst colleagues (Montgomery 1992). Thankfully, this type of legal distortion is relatively rare, and in most cases the law supports rather than frustrates team working. Professionals should therefore challenge suggestions that the law is a barrier to good multidisciplinary practice to ensure that they are not merely being used as an excuse to constrain progress.

This chapter considers the legal context in which the multidisciplinary team operates. It begins by outlining three concepts around which the analysis is organized: responsibility, accountability and liability. It then examines the legal principles that govern teamwork in palliative care using these concepts as a framework.

## Concepts

The three concepts of responsibility, accountability and liability overlap in terms of the circumstances in which they apply but capture different aspects of the workings of a team. Responsibility is used here as a broad concept describing the actions with which and people for whom members of the team should be concerned. It is as much an ethical as legal issue, but occasionally the question '*who* is responsible' for something is important in identifying the member of the team whose role it is to resolve problems. In this sense, responsibility for something may also be linked to authority to determine what should be done. Accountability is used to cover the processes by which members of the team can be 'called to account', i.e. required to explain their actions to others, with the possibility of some form of sanction being administered if the explanation is unsatisfactory. They may feel responsible for things without being exposed to such formal accountability, for example where a mishap occurs by chance unrelated to any error or misjudgement. Liability looks at legal channels of accountability. Here the 'victim' of a mishap can seek some form of redress, typically compensation. Society may also impose sanctions on those who break the criminal law. The section on liability is concerned with who bears the legal consequences of a finding that expected standards have not been met.

## Responsibility

Mutual responsibility is an important bond in teams. Team working involves a sense of common purpose in which the members of an effective team hold a collective responsibility for the patients in their care, independent of individual roles. In this sense, if something is unsatisfactory, everyone may feel responsible because it represents a failure of the team. Equally, colleagues may recognize a responsibility to put things right even where they have not caused the difficulties. In this sense, responsibility captures something much broader than any legal obligation. Strong teams are likely to have a well-developed sense of mutual responsibility. However, no accountability or liability would follow from this feeling of responsibility because it provides only an emotional or perhaps sometimes moral, rather than legally recognized, obligation.

Complexities in the concept of responsibility may arise in a number of respects. One concerns the people for whom the team is responsible. Clearly, the team will be responsible for their care of the patient, but are they also responsible for the patient's relatives? The law has traditionally sought to limit the scope of those for whom we can be held responsible by two main techniques. The first concerns the directness of the relationship between the parties. Unless there is reasonable proximity between them, then it would be seen as unjust to hold the team responsible for their welfare in law. This is sometimes described as the question of to whom we hold a duty of care. The second concerns the priority of duties. Here we may have a duty of care to (responsibility for) someone but the implications are outweighed by a higher duty. Thus, we may have a responsibility towards carers to help them deal with the death of someone that they love, and this would point to sharing information about the patient's prognosis. However, that duty to the carers is outweighed by the patient's right to confidentiality unless they have waived it by giving their consent to the disclosure. Thus, there is not liability to relatives for distress caused by refusing to disclose information without the patient's agreement.

A second complexity concerns the relationship between responsibility and authority. Asserting that something is 'my responsibility' can be a mechanism for excluding others from it: it is mine and not yours. In this context, the allocation of responsibility is a mechanism for giving people the authority to act. This may be important to clarify roles, so that it is clear who is responsible for a task in order to ensure that someone takes it on and gets it done. It may relate to the management of risk—ensuring that only those with the training or experience for dealing with issues are permitted to address them. It is in this sense that responsibility for prescribing certain drugs is limited to specific categories or professionals. Similarly, employers may require specific training before certain tasks are taken on. This is perhaps best captured using the concept of demarcation explored later.

## Accountability

Two crucial questions will arise in relation to accountability within teams. The first concerns which aspects of the work of the team individual members are accountable for. This will depend on how tasks are allocated within the team. The second question concerns the processes of accountability. These will differ for team members according to their profession and employer, and is dealt with in the second section of the chapter. The first question merits further explanation here.

Three different type of relationship may arise in the workings of a team. The implications of each for accountability will be different. The first type of relationship is *delegation*. In delegation, accountability is retained by the person delegating a task or responsibility but the work will actually be carried out by someone else on their behalf. In this situation, responsibility and accountability will be shared by both the person delegating (the delegator) and the person to whom the task is delegated. The role is seen as properly sitting with the delegator, but one that can sometimes be entrusted to another. Should a mishap occur, both the person delegating a task and the person carrying it out will be called to account, although the tests applied to see whether they have practised properly may be slightly different according to the post that they hold (see below).

The second type of relationship is *demarcation*. Here separate roles are defined. Members of the team will be accountable for their own roles, but not for something that happens outside of the scope of their responsibilities. Should a mishap occur, the first issue to be resolved would be to identify what went wrong and whose actions led to the problem. From this, it would become apparent which member of the team should be held to account. Others will not be held to account because the error was not made in their sphere of responsibility. This type of relationship sees the work of the team as a series of parallel roles that are separable and allocated to different individual members. Difficulties in carrying out one of these roles are seen as a problem for the individual whose role it is but not that of other team members. Although they may feel a mutual sense of responsibility, they would not be held to account for their colleague's failure because it is separate from their own sphere of accountability.

The third type of relationship is *referral*. Here accountability is transferred from one person to another. Unlike delegation, where one team member properly refers an issue to another they divest themselves of further accountability by the act of referral. Unlike demarcation, accountability is not escaped because the role belonged to someone else, but because responsibility has been reallocated to a colleague through a clear referral process. Whether or not referral has been effective in transferring accountability will usually be resolved by examining the process.

The difference between demarcation and referral will be particularly important where a mishap occurs because of an omission rather than an action. Demarcation of roles will enable the person who should have acted to be readily identified. Without it, it may be impossible to determine which member of a team should be held to account because it will not be clear whose responsibility it was to act. In such circumstances, recourse may also be had to the principle that liability needs to be fixed for the overall failure of the team to provide the required standard of care rather than calling individuals to account.

### Liability

While responsibility may be moral as well as legal, and accountability may utilize a range of mechanisms beyond court processes, liability is specifically a legal doctrine. It is used to denote the possibility of judicial sanctions being visited on someone who has breached the required legal standards. Liability is therefore used here to describe the situations where health professionals may find themselves acting illegally (contrary to a criminal rule) or unlawfully (without legal justification, such as without the requisite consent) or in breach of the legal standards of care (as in malpractice litigation where the team member does something that is in itself lawful but which they do so badly that patients are entitled to compensation if they suffer injury as a result of the error).

Where the standards are established in the criminal law, then the likely sanction will be punishment (usually in the form of a fine or imprisonment).

Here, the fundamental principle is that a wrong has been committed against society not against individuals. Even where the 'victim' is willing (such as in voluntary euthanasia), the law will regard the breach of the criminal law as punishable. In practice, in England and Wales, the decision whether to prosecute alleged breaches of the criminal law will be taken by the Crown Prosecution Service (CPS).

Prosecutors decide whether they should bring cases by considering whether the evidence of an offence is strong enough to secure a conviction and whether it is in the public interest to prosecute. It may therefore be that an apparent offence, such as homicide (which is how active euthanasia would currently be defined), might not result in a prosecution because it was not clear what happened. Thus, in the Nigel Cox case, there was no murder prosecution because the body had been cremated so that the cause of death could not be ascertained. Consequently, it was not clear whether the drugs Dr Cox had administered had in fact killed the patient in question. Instead the doctor was prosecuted for attempted murder on the basis that it was not necessary to determine whether the attempt was successful to prove that offence [*R v Cox* (1992) 12 BMLR 38, see below for further discussion]. Occasionally, the CPS might decide that there is no public benefit in a prosecution. An example might be a 'mercy killing' by a family member where there is no hint that the relative had anything other than the deceased's best interest at heart.

In the palliative care context, liability in criminal law is almost always personal. Key issues arise in relation to teams as to whether relying on colleagues creates a risk of exposure to prosecution. This is discussed below in terms of the relevance of 'following instructions' as a defence and in terms of the possibility that someone could be found to be an 'accessory' to an offence committed by someone else. There is also a possibility that organizations can be corporately guilty of offences. In at least one case, an NHS Trust has pleaded guilty to offences under health and safety legislation on the basis that poor training and supervision of junior doctors had led to an unsafe system of practice that resulted in a patient dying when this could have been avoided. This criminal liability was visited on the Trust, not individuals personally responsible for the supervision of the staff concerned. Thus, a failure of employers to establish proper systems for safe working (including team working) may give rise to corporate criminal liability.

The other main category of liability is usually described by lawyers as 'civil'. It refers to the obligations owed by members of society to each other, not to the relationship between society and its members. Here the sanction will normally be monetary compensation rather than punishment. Further, the 'victim' is entitled to choose whether or not to exercise their rights to sue. Thus, there may be circumstances in which the potential for legal liability exists, but patients do not sue. Within the NHS, malpractice litigation is no longer managed in a way that exposes individual team members to risk.

Rather, through a system known as NHS indemnity, the Service bears the financial cost of claims. In the private or not-for-profit sector, the position will be slightly different. Primary legal liability will lie with individual team members for their personal mistakes. However, where they are employees, their employer will also be liable for those mistakes under the legal doctrine known as 'vicarious liability'.

Patients who believe they have been the victims of negligence will usually sue the employer not the individual member of the team, as it is more likely that the employer can afford to pay any damages that might be ordered than that an individual could do so. In strict legal theory, the employer could then seek reimbursement of the money paid out from an employee, but this is highly unlikely in practice. It is also possible that courts will need to consider how liability is to be apportioned between members of the team in proportion to their responsibility for the patient's injuries (see Montgomery 2003, pp. 201–202)

## Principles of malpractice law

The basic principle of the law of clinical negligence, usually thought of by health professionals as malpractice litigation, is that patients who suffer injury as a result of the carelessness, or substandard care, of the people caring for them should receive monetary compensation. This principle is not peculiar to health care—it is the same basic principle that leads to a car driver who has caused an accident being made to pay for the damage to the victims' cars. Where professional activities are concerned, the courts have recognized that a high degree of expertise may be involved and have been reluctant to criticize practice unless it is clear that it has been unacceptable.

The test that has been developed to establish whether professionals have fallen below the required legal standards is know as the *Bolam* test, after the case in which it was formulated. The judge in that case said:

A doctor is not guilty of negligence if he has acted in accordance with a practice accepted as proper by a responsible body of medical men skilled in that particular art [*Bolam* v *Friern HMC* [1957] 2 All ER 118, 121].

It can be seen that the essence of this test is that it is based on 'peer review' of professional colleagues. Compliance with an acceptable practice, as judged by responsible colleagues, is a sufficient answer to an allegation of negligence. It is important to note that there may be more than one acceptable practice, so that the court is not required to select the best practice when there is divergence of views amongst professionals [*Maynard* v. *W. Midlands RHA* [1985] 1 All ER 635]. In general, this means that following prevailing professional wisdom will be a sufficient protection from a negligence allegation. Only where that practice has no logical basis are the courts likely to take a different view [*Bolitho* v *Hackney HA* [1997] 4 All ER 771].

It should also be noted that the test requires the courts to identify the appropriate comparators for acceptable standards by reference to the speciality in which care is being given (in the words of the judge, 'that particular art'). Thus to assess an accusation that there has been negligence by members of a palliative care team, it would be necessary to obtain evidence of what was acceptable from responsible palliative care professionals.

The most important judicial decision for understanding how this basic principle applies to health care teams is not a palliative care case. It concerned a little boy called Martin Wilsher who had been cared for in a neonatal intensive care unit. By the end of his stay, Martin was nearly blind, suffering from a condition called retrolental fibroplasia. This condition can be caused by excessive oxygen in the bloodstream and Martin had been given extra oxygen during his care. On Martin's behalf, his mother sued the health authority for damages, claiming that there had been a negligent mistake that had caused Martin's blindness. The case was taken all the way to the House of Lords in relation to the precise legal test of causation—how certain did the proof that the extra oxygen caused the blindness need to be before the health authority would be ordered to pay compensation. On this point, it was found that it must be more likely than not that it was the cause [*Wilsher* v *Essex AHA* [1988] 1 All ER 871, HL].

More importantly for this chapter, there was considerable discussion of the application of the law to different team members as a result of the circumstances surrounding Martin's care. The evidence showed that there had clearly been mistakes in assessing Martin's needs that had resulted in him being given additional oxygen inappropriately. The circumstances of these mistakes and the judicial analysis of their significance are very important for understanding the application of the principles of negligence to health care teams. This analysis can be found in the judgements in the Court of Appeal, which were not challenged in the House of Lords [*Wilsher* v *Essex AHA* [1986] 3 All ER 801].

Martin had been born prematurely, very floppy and blue. He had difficulties breathing. He was taken to the special care baby unit and his colour improved with the help of oxygen administered through a mask. The senior house officer (SHO) on duty set in place the usual procedures for monitoring a baby in this condition, including the use of an arterial catheter to enable readings of Martin's oxygen levels. Unfortunately, the SHO inadvertently inserted the catheter into a vein instead of an artery. This error was not found to be negligent. The severed ends of the vessels in the umbilical stump were difficult to identify, and competent doctors could mistake them. Thus, inserting the catheter into the wrong vessel was not negligent in law, even though it was a clinical error.

It was clear from the lack of consistency between the oxygen readings and other observations that there was something wrong with the monitoring. The

189

SHO responded to this by arranging an X-ray and asking the registrar to look at it. As a result, the catheter was removed and a new one inserted, but unfortunately the same error was made. It was not identified despite further X-rays. Only later when additional readings of arterial blood were taken via a different route did the cause of the error become apparent and the oxygenation reduced.

This was not, therefore, a case of a single error but a failure of the team as a whole to ensure the proper level of care. The SHO had identified concerns and sought the registrar's opinion. Nursing staff would also have been involved in observing the baby. It was known that something was amiss, but it took some time to identify the problem. The court had to consider how liability should be assessed in such cases of imperfect care. The solution was to recognize that each 'post' within the team carried different expectations. This was not an issue of the qualifications or experience of the individual, nor of 'rank' or 'status'. The standard of care was not related to what was expected of the rank of SHO, but of the post of SHO in a specialist baby care unit. Similarly, had the issue concerned the practice of a nurse, it would not be his or her profession that determined the standard expected, but the post of staff nurse on such a unit.

Applying this approach, the Court of Appeal found that the SHO was not negligent. The insertion of the catheter into a vein was not negligent, because it was a mistake that could have been made by a competent doctor. Given his post in the team, the failure of the SHO to identify from the X-ray that the catheter had been misplaced was not negligent. A competent doctor holding that post could have made that error. When it became apparent that something was amiss, the SHO had acted responsibly by referring the situation to the registrar for a more experienced opinion. Errors were made, but they did not involve falling below the standard expected from an SHO on a special care baby unit. The post of SHO was necessarily one in which the doctor would have limited experience. That is why the post is supervised. However, the registrar was found to be negligent. He held a more senior post, which carried with it a higher expectation of expertise and experience. The error was not one that a competent registrar would have made.

The *Wilsher* case indicates some important principles of liability in respect of multidisciplinary teams. First, the standard of care that people are expected to reach will be tailored to their post in the team. Members of specialist teams such as those in palliative care will be judged against the standards of their colleagues in that speciality. Posts will vary between different teams, depending on how they are organized, and it may be necessary to understand the demarcation of roles carefully to determine precisely what the demands of the post would be. Secondly, drawing on the support of colleagues may serve to repair otherwise substandard practice. Thus, the SHO protected himself from a finding of negligence by referring the case to the registrar. Team members are expected to recognize their limitations, and a failure to do so when all responsible practitioners would expect it could in itself be negligent.

Thirdly, the Court of Appeal specifically rejected the suggestion that there could be a 'team' liability principle whereby each of the members of a team held themselves out as capable of undertaking all the procedures that the team as a whole set out to perform. This would have been highly unsatisfactory, as it would have exposed a junior nurse to litigation for failure to possess the skills and experience of a medical consultant. Had it been accepted, it would have undermined the development of effective teams because it would have required members to live up to impossible standards. By fixing the standard of care according to the post that people take within the team, the law reinforces the mutual interdependence that characterizes good teamwork.

Although not relevant in the *Wilsher* case, it should also be noted that English law has rejected another possible legal principle that would have served to undermine good team working. That is the 'captain of the ship' doctrine, which seeks to fix liability for any mistakes made by team members on the leader of the team. Thus, if the person responsible for leading the team was a medical consultant, this doctrine would have made them liable for compensation for mistakes made by other members of staff, whether or not they were personally involved. This would also distort the dynamics of successful teams by requiring a hierarchical structure.

*Wilsher* also examined a different liability principle, which has become more widespread in practice. That is known as 'direct liability'. Under this principle, rather than asking about the conduct of individual members of the team, the focus is on whether the organization has delivered the care that patients are entitled to expect. On this basis, the question is not whether any individual has made a mistake, but whether the overall quality of care meets acceptable standards. Thus a badly organized hospice could be sued if the organization failures caused harm to a patient [see *Bull* v *Devon AHA* [1993] 4 Med. LR 117 for an example concerning maternity services]. This approach serves to protect patients by making compensation available while reducing the scrutiny of individual team members in favour of considering the effectiveness of the team as a whole.

## Death, dying and the law

The main area of criminal law that is relevant to palliative care concerns decisions that might lead to a patient dying earlier than would otherwise occur. This will typically be where a decision is made to refrain from attempting curative treatment in favour of palliation in the interests of the patient's dignity and according to their wishes. It is clear that competent patients are entitled to reject curative treatment so, when this is the result of the patient's choice, no liability, criminal or civil, will arise. Things are a little more complicated where the patient has not made a choice and is no longer competent to do so. Here the professionals must act in the patient's best interests. In cases where there is uncertainty over whether those interests point to withholding a particular treatment, the legal test to be applied to assess whether the professional judgement is acceptable is the *Bolam* test, discussed above. The House of Lords has held that this is the case even where one consequence of the choice of treatment could be that the patient is allowed to die from their underlying health condition [*Airedale NHS Trust* v *Bland* [1993] 1 All ER 821, see Montgomery 2003, Chapter 20 for discussion of this case and others in this section]. Failure to save life could in principle constitute homicide if there is a duty to act, but there will only be such a duty where all responsible health professionals would keep the patient alive.

The position is different where members of the team take steps that will actually cause the patient's earlier death, as in active euthanasia. Here the basic principle is that actions that cause the death of the patient will constitute homicide. Even where there is an active step that may have shortened a patient's life health, such as the administration of medicine, professionals may not be acting illegally. This is important in order to protect palliative care professionals from unfair accusations of murder where the use of pain-relieving drugs is suspected of leading to the death of a patient.

There is an acceptance that no crime is committed by a health professional where three circumstances exist.

- First, that the patient was already close to death (so that the death could be said to have been natural, not caused by the medication).
- Secondly, where the medicine given was acceptable professional practice (probably as judged by peer review).
- Thirdly, where there was no ulterior motive, so that the purpose of administration was to achieve the comfort of the patient, not their death [*R* v *Adams* (1957) Crim LR 365; *R* v *Moor* (2000) Crim LR 31, 41, 566].

The principal perpetrator of offences of this sort would be the people who took the decision to withdraw treatment in order to kill a patient, who administered the drug or who took the steps that caused the death (such as smothering the patient). Team members could conceivably commit these criminal offences as accessories if they incited, aided or abetted the perpetrator. Such accessories are just as guilty of the crime, although they might receive a lighter sentence. Clearly, given the philosophy of palliative care, this is unlikely to occur in well-functioning teams.

The accessory principle can be seen most clearly in the specific offence of assisting suicide, where it has been codified in section 2 of the Suicide Act 1961. This offence is committed where 'a person aids, abets, counsels or procures the suicide of another, or an attempt by another to commit suicide'. Case law has established that three things have to be shown to prove that an offence has been committed: (1) that the accused knew that suicide was contemplated; (2) that he or she approved or assented to it; and (3) that he or she encouraged the suicide attempt. Giving someone pills saying that they should be taken to end his or her life would be an offence. So, too, would putting people in touch with someone you know will help them end their lives [*R* v *McShane* (1977) 66 Cr. App. R. 97; *R* v *Reed* (1982) Crim. LR 819; *A.G.* v *Able* [1984] 1 All ER 277]. It is this rule that makes physician-assisted suicide illegal. Again, given the philosophy of palliative care, this will not occur in functional teams.

The implications of these rules for palliative care teams are best illustrated by a case study on concerns over the use of drugs. This will form the conclusion of this chapter so that the interplay of criminal and civil law can be explored. That will show how criminal liability cannot easily be avoided by reliance on colleagues, while trust in the judgement of colleagues may be sufficient where civil litigation is concerned.

## Professional accountability

Registered professionals are subject to disciplinary procedures before their regulatory bodies, which are concerned to ensure that the public is protected against unsafe practitioners. Where necessary, a finding of professional misconduct can lead to the practitioner's licence to practise being removed. This avenue of accountability is only relevant to professionals and will not cover lay members of the team or family carers. Nevertheless, the standards established by the professional bodies are a helpful guide to expectations of good practice in health care.

The regulatory bodies for health professionals now recognize that multi-disciplinary team working is now the norm rather than the exception. The General Medical Council (2001) document *Good Medical Practice* notes.

36. Healthcare is increasingly provided by multi-disciplinary teams. Working in a team does not change your personal accountability for your professional conduct and the care you provide. When working in a team, you must:

- respect the skills and contributions of your colleagues;
- maintain professional relationships with patients;
- communicate effectively with colleagues within and outside the team;
- make sure that your patients and colleagues understand your professional status and specialty, your role and responsibilities in the team and who is responsible for each aspect of patients' care;
- participate in regular reviews and audit of the standards and performance of the team, taking steps to remedy any deficiencies;
- be willing to deal openly and supportively with problems in the performance, conduct or health of team members.

The Nursing and Midwifery Council (2004) similarly instructs nurses and midwives in its *Code of Professional Conduct* that

4.2 You are expected to work co-operatively within teams and to respect the skills, expertise and contributions of your colleagues. You must treat them fairly and without discrimination.

4.3 You must communicate effectively and share your knowledge, skill and expertise with other members of the team as required for the benefit of patients and clients.

Recognition of the importance of teamwork does not preclude some important dimensions of professional acountability that require discussion here. First, the principle that professionals remain accountable for their personal practice when they work in teams. Thus, like the General Medical Council (GMC), the Nursing and Midwifery Council (NMC) identifies that personal accountability is not removed by membership of a team:

4.5 When working as a member of a team, you remain accountable for your professional conduct, any care you provide and any omission on your part.

This professional accountability is in addition to the possibility of legal liability and obligations as employees.

Secondly, the tendency is for professional groups to protect their traditional roles rather than promote flexibility in the interests of patient care. The GMC guidance quoted above encourages doctors to ensure that patients and colleagues understand the professional status of doctors. The NMC Code implies grudging acceptance of other professional and lay roles when it states

4.6 You may be expected to delegate care delivery to others who are not registered nurses or midwives. Such delegation must not compromise existing care but must be directed to meeting the needs and serving the interests of patients and clients. You remain accountable for the appropriateness of the delegation, for ensuring that the person who does the work is able to do it and that adequate supervision or support is provided.

However, it should be noted that the NMC Code also explicitly notes that the health care team should be given a broad definition:

4.1 The team includes the patient or client, the patient's or client's family, informal carers and health and social care professionals in the National Health Service, independent and voluntary sectors.

In well-functioning teams, protective attitudes to professional status and roles will not play a significant role. There are very few activities that are limited to particular professions by law rather than by custom and practice. Where things are merely customary, they can be varied by agreement between the team. Only where the law limits powers and functions to those with specific professional status (such as the prescription of certain medicines or the certification of death) are the boundaries strict. The only significant examples of this in the palliative care context concern the prescription of certain medicines (which is restricted in law to doctors and certain other specifically licensed professionals) and the certification of death (a medical monopoly). There is no restriction on the administration of medicines, although patient safety concerns will usually give rise to local policies on who should administer medicines, with safeguards against errors.

The third area in which professional guidance is helpful is in drawing attention to important facets of successful teams. In the GMC document *Management for Doctors* issued in Feburary 2006, it is noted that problems can arise when communication is poor or there is lack of clarity over responsibilities. Thus, it is recommended that team leaders

- make sure that colleagues understand the professional status and specialty of all team members, their roles and responsibilities in the team, and who is responsible for each aspect of patient care
- make sure that staff are clear about their individual and team objectives, their personal and collective responsibilities for patient and public safety, and for openly and honestly recording and discussing problems (para 50)

The document expects that the skills and contributions of colleagues are respected and that 'all team members have an opportunity to contribute to discussions and that they understand and accept the decisions taken'. This guidance stresses the importance of clear demarcation of roles within the team together with understanding of common responsibilities and objectives.

Turning to communication, the GMC document expects medical managers to

- communicate effectively with colleagues within and outside the team; you should make sure that arrangements are in place for relevant information to be passed on to the team promptly

One important aspect of communication concerns the scope of confidentiality and the position of carers and lay members of the team. Although confidentiality is a professional obligation and is enforced by the professional regulatory bodies, it is based on respect for the privacy and autonomy of patients. The principal justification for sharing confidential information is the consent of the patient. It is generally expected that patients are happy for information to be shared within the health care team, and this seems to be supported by research into public expectations (Consumers' Association, NHS Information Authority and Health Which? 2002). There is less certainty about the extent to which patients appreciate that social workers and chaplains may also need to be party to confidential information. Two steps are advisable to ensure that confidentiality requirements are met. The first is that all those with whom confidential information is to be shared are bound by their employment contract to keep confidential information secret. The second is to explain to patients how information is shared within the team and obtain their consent to that approach. This also provides an opportunity to establish which family members can be given confidential information.

Finally, the GMC document *Good Medical Practice* contains a concise statement of good practice in delegation and referral:

46. Delegation involves asking a nurse, doctor, medical student or other health care worker to provide treatment or care on your behalf. When you delegate care or treatment you must be sure that the person to whom you delegate is competent to carry out the procedure or provide the therapy involved. You must always pass on enough information about the patient and the treatment needed. You will still be responsible for the overall management of the patient.

47. Referral involves transferring some or all of the responsibility for the patient's care, usually temporarily and for a particular purpose, such as additional investigation, care or treatment, which falls outside your competence. Usually you will refer patients to another registered medical practitioner. If this is not the case, you must be satisfied that any health care professional to whom you refer a patient is accountable to a statutory regulatory body, and that a registered medical practitioner, usually a general practitioner, retains overall responsibility for the management of the patient.

It should be borne in mind that for aspects of the team's work that do not need to be carried out by a registered health professional, there is no reason in principle why delegation or referral should be limited to passing work to other professionals. In such cases of referral, it would be important to clarify that some form of accountability is in place, such as to an employer.

## Employment obligations

The principle of vicarious liability and the practical workings of negligence litigation provide considerable comfort to employees from exposure to legal liability. Being an employee also brings with it certain expectations of conformity with the employer's way of doing things, including the operation of teams providing care. All employees are expected to follow the 'lawful and reasonable' instructions of their employer. This is reinforced through employment law, in that failure to follow such instructions could lead to disciplinary action, even to the extent of dismissal in extreme cases. Clearly, this has important implications for team working in palliative care.

Employers are entitled to establish a philosophy of care, protocols and procedures, and determine the demarcation of responsibilities within their workforce. These could include hierarchical demarcations such as leadership responsibilities. They may determine who has primary responsibilities for aspects of the work and whether or not they can delegate it. They may also establish referral procedures for transferring responsibilities; ranging from the regular hand-over at the end of a shift to decisions about admission to units.

In a well-functioning team, such arrangements help ensure that effort is not wasted and care is not compromised by confusion over roles. Occasionally, however, difficulties may arise and employers' instructions may be challenged. Very occasionally, matters escalate and reach the legal sphere. This happened in one mental health nursing case, which illuminated the sort of distinction that industrial tribunals would make when considering how individual clinical accountability and obligations to follow reasonable instructions may conflict.

The case concerned a nurse who disapproved of electroconvulsive therapy (ECT) and sought to ensure that a patient in his care did not receive it by refusing to cooperate with the treatment. He was dismissed by his employer for refusing to follow the agreed procedures. That dismissal was upheld by the Court of Appeal, on the basis that he had an implied contractual duty as an employee to follow reasonable instructions [*Owen* v *Coventry HA* (1986), 19 December, unreported]. The fact that he disapproved of the unit's use of ECT and the clinical judgement of medical colleagues that it was appropriate for his patient did not entitle him to refuse to participate in the treatment. The Court of Appeal did indicate that there might be circumstances when the obligation to follow instructions could be over-ridden by a team member's obligation to act in the best interests of the patient. This might be so where there are specific circumstances, that had not already been assessed, that made the treatment contraindicated. However, the nurse in question had not shown that this was the case. Instead, he was refusing to accept the employer's clinical policy permitting the use of ECT and the demarcation of responsibility under which the doctors were expected to determine when it should be used.

It is of course perfectly proper for team members to challenge policies that they believe are misguided. However, there is a time and place to do so and it will not usually be appropriate to raise these issues while providing care to individual patients. Employers and team members are entitled to expect that colleagues can be relied upon to follow agreed procedures. Without such reassurance, the benefits of teams cannot be realized. The employment obligation to follow employers' instructions is the working through of this principle in the legal context. It enables duplication of effort to be avoided and consistency of care to be maintained.

The obligations of employees to follow agreed procedures can also provide a mechanism for securing best practice within a team. While legal liability in negligence aims to ensure that minimum standards are not breached, it offers little incentive to improve practice beyond those standards. Accountability as employees and professionals is concerned with more than basic standards of care.

## Conclusion: a case study

A useful case study for the respective liabilities of team members can be seen in the context of inappropriate usage of drugs in palliative care. Consider the situation where a doctor writes up a large dose of a prescription-only painkilling drug and a nurse is concerned that it is not appropriate. In this case, two very different areas of law might come into play.

It could be that the use of the drug would breach the criminal law of homicide. This would happen if the administration would cause the early death of the patient and the special defence of appropriate palliative care could not be established. In those circumstances, both the doctor prescribing the drug and the person administering it would be guilty of murder. In the context of the criminal law, following instructions is no excuse from liability. If the nurse had any reason to believe that the death was being caused improperly, then she or he would need to refuse to participate in order to avoid criminal liability. The nurse cannot avoid personal responsibility.

The situation would be different if the nurse did not anticipate that the consequence of the apparently excessive dose would be the patient's early death. Here the legal question would concern negligence, or malpractice. There is a clear demarcation of responsibility in law, with the task of deciding whether the drug is appropriate, and at what dosage, sitting with the prescriber. Faced with a prescription that appears inappropriate, other team members are expected to challenge the instructions [see *Hillyer* v *St Bartholemew's Hospital* [1909] 2 KB 820, concerning a nurse, and *Dwyer* v *Roderick* (1983) 127 SJ 806, concerning a pharmacist]. If they were to fail to do so, they would be failing in their professional duties and would therefore be negligent. If the patient suffered injury as a result, then they would be liable in negligence to pay compensation (along with the doctor).

If the doctor's instructions were challenged by another team member but confirmed as unchanged, then the law would usually accept reliance on the skill of the doctor as a reasonable step for the others to take. Consequently, if it turned out that the doctor's judgement was negligent and the patient was harmed, only the doctor (and their employer under vicarious liability) would be liable to pay compensation. In this context, deferring to the expertise of the doctor would be a protection for the other members of the team. Their obligations to the patient to protect them from mishap would be exhausted by the challenge made to the decision. Professional regulatory bodies might go further, and nurses are advised to refuse to administer medicines that they think are inappropriate. However, the law would regard following confirmed instructions from the appropriate decision maker as sufficient to meet the required standard of care. The Wilsher case, discussed above, indicates that this principle does not depend on the legal demarcation in relation to prescriptions, but rather depends on clarity of roles and hierarchies within the team.

This protection is not absolute, however, and there may be circumstances where following instructions would not constitute an adequate answer to malpractice litigation. This is because responsible professionals will not always regard it as acceptable to accept grossly inappropriate decisions from their colleagues. If when instructions are being followed it becomes apparent that they are clearly inconsistent with observable facts, then professionals would be expected to take remedial action [*Tanswell* v *Nelson* (1959) *Times*, 11 Feb; CLY 2254]. Mere suspicion that instructions were 'unsuitable and improper' is not sufficient, that would merely trigger the obligation to challenge instructions, but where they were 'manifestly wrong' then professionals would not be expected to follow them [*Junor* v *McNichol* (1959) *Times*, 26 March].

Thus, much would depend on the nature of the concerns about a colleague's instructions. If the prescription is for a drug, or combination of drugs that would seem to have no proper purpose and would be likely to cause the patient's death, then other team members would have little choice. If they were to cooperate with the administration of the drugs, then they would risk being guilty of murder. Their professional responsibilities to protect the interests of their patients would require them to act to ensure that the proposed plan of care did not go ahead without scrutiny. Their clinical governance responsibilities as employees would raise a similar obligation to report their concerns so as to assure the quality and safety of care given. This would seem to be the situation in a case such as that of Nigel Cox, a rheumatologist working in Winchester in 1992 who administered a lethal dose of potassium chloride. Expert evidence indicated that the drug had no pain-relieving qualities, suggesting that it was intended to end life rather than control distress. The jury convicted Dr Cox of attempted murder [*R* v *Cox* (1992) 12 BMLR 38]. The case came to light because a nurse recognized that the drug appeared inappropriate and raised her concerns—something she was clearly obliged to do.

Contrast the situation where the prescription was of an unusually high dosage of morphine. Here, it would be less clear that the intention was to cause death. Juries have acquitted doctors in the past where prosecutors have alleged that high dosages of morphine had been used deliberately to cause death but doctors claimed to be acting in order to relieve pain and suffering [e.g. *R* v *Adams* [1957] Crim LR 365; *R* v *Moor* [2000] Crim LR 31, 41, 566]. If juries are uncertain, even after hearing all the evidence presented in a forensic context, then it is probably reasonable for team members to accept instructions on high dosages, provided they challenge them to ensure they were what the doctor intended. Only if they were 'manifestly wrong' need they take further steps.

Most concerns within multiprofessional teams will be over less dramatic circumstances, and the general principle remains that colleagues are entitled to rely on each other's judgements. However, it is hoped that this case study helps illustrate when that normal position is superseded by additional consid-erations. Well-functioning palliative care teams will find that liability rules generally reflect their collective responsibilities, respect their demarcation of different roles when appropriate, and provide a structure within which careful referral and delegation not only enhances patient care but protects members from allegations of malpractice.

## References

Consumers'Association, NHS Information Authority and Health Which? (2002). *Share with Care! People's Views on Consent and Confidentiality or Patient Information—Qualitative and Quantitative Research: Final Report.* Consumers' Association in association with NHS Information Authority and Health Which?, London.

General Medical Council (2001). *Good Medical Practice,* 3rd edn. GMC, London.

General Medical Council (2006). *Management for Doctors.* GMC, London.

Montgomery J (1992). 'Doctors' handmaidens: the legal contribution'. In: McVeigh S and Wheeler S, ed. *Law, Health and Medical Regulation.* Dartmouth, Aldershot, UK, pp. 141–168.

Montgomery J (2003). *Health Care Law,* 2nd edn. Oxford University Press, Oxford.

Nursing and Midwifery Council (2004). *Code of Professional Conduct: Standards for Conduct, Performance and Ethics.* NMC, London.

# 13

# Team effectiveness

*Barbara Monroe and Peter Speck*

## Introduction

*Peter Speck*

In the course of planning this textbook, and discussing the content with the other authors, I have found myself returning to two questions. Are teams the best way of providing a service and how do we know if they are effective? These questions may seem to run counter to the main text, but I feel it important to face them if the book is to be relevant to the 'efficacy-demanding' culture within which we offer palliative care.

In *A First Class Service*, the Department of Health strongly recommend that more attention be paid to improving teamwork between professionals (Department of Health 1998). The NICE guidance (2004) also advocates team working as the most beneficial model, and in the course of this book we have explored the many facets that come into play during creating, developing and sustaining a healthy multi- or interdisciplinary team. However, it has nagged away at me that it is difficult to identify much empirical evidence that such a team is always the best way to provide good patient care. The sparse nature of the evidence in relation to the benefits of nurse–doctor collaboration has also been commented on by Zwarenstein and Reeves (2000) in a *British Medical Journal* editorial. While they conclude that there are one or two trials that seem to indicate a worthwhile benefit from working together, they also highlight that problems in collaboration are widespread and common (Zwarenstein and Bryant 2000).

An early study by Ellershaw *et al.* (1995) looked at the effectiveness of a hospital palliative care team. The team is described as 'part of the pain relief team and works in an advisory capacity. Team medical and nursing expertise is combined with support from other disciplines as appropriate' (p. 146). This was a prospective study looking at 125 hospital in-patients with malignant disease referred to a 'hospital advisory palliative care team'. They conclude that the team was effective at improving symptom control, facilitating the understanding of the diagnosis and prognosis, and contributing to the appropriate transfer of patients to home, a hospice or another hospital. It is not clear from this study, however, whether the outcome benefits were due to effective team working by the palliative care team (whose role was advisory) or to the ward clinical team achieving better decision making because of access to a specialist resource that could have been provided by a skilled individual rather than a team.

A systematic review undertaken by Hearn and Higginson (1998) looked specifically at palliative care interventions and found that there were significant improvement in outcomes for those cared for by a specialist palliative care team over those receiving standard care. They reviewed 18 studies, including five randomized controlled trials, and found that specialist teams were effective in improving satisfaction and identifying and dealing with more patient and family needs. They also identified that multiprofessional approaches to palliative care reduced the overall cost of care because they reduced the amount of time patients spent within an expensive hospital setting. The improved outcomes for patients included more time spent at home, greater satisfaction for patients and carers, better symptom control and greater likelihood of patients dying where they wished to. Many of the outcome measures used in these studies related to pain and symptom relief, days spent in hospital or at home, and comparative costs of home versus hospital care. It remains difficult to get a picture of what the 'unique' contribution of the team itself might be and therefore to obtain answers to my two questions: are teams the best way to provide care, and are they more effective?

I discussed these questions with Barbara Monroe, Chief Executive at St Christopher's Hospice, as someone who has had a lifetime of working within, and leading, teams with both a single and a multidisciplinary structure. Initially we felt it should not be too difficult to assent to the commonly held view that teams are the best way to ensure that seamless quality service which specialist palliative care wishes to provide. As our discussions continued, we recognized, as indicated above, that there was not a great deal of empirical evidence to support the view that an interdisciplinary team always improved care for the patient. The following reflection, contributed by Barbara, captures in her own words the main threads of the discussions which I and others had with Barbara as she sought to answer my questions and highlight some important issues for teamwork in the future against a background of further organizational change in health care.

# Team effectiveness—a reflection

*Barbara Monroe*

The necessity for, and utility of, multidisciplinary teams in palliative care has become an almost automatic assumption. The assumption stems from an understanding of the need to integrate and coordinate the multiple skills and complex knowledge base required to deliver the holistic care to which palliative care aspires. It also contains echoes of the in-patient roots of hospice care and the enthusiasm for therapeutic 'communities' evident in many of the health and social care innovations of the 1960s (Clark 2002). The issue of measuring the effectiveness of multiprofessional teams in delivering palliative care is a fascinating one. A review of the literature suggests that it is a question that has never really been addressed. Although Gysels and Higginson's extensive review of outcome evidence in the National Institute of Clinical Excellence Report on *Improving Supportive and Palliative Care for Adults with Cancer* (2004) finds that 'the evidence strongly supports specialist palliative care teams..... as a means of improving outcomes for cancer patients', an examination of the literature studied suggests that the evidence supports specialist palliative care input as a means of improving some outcomes, rather than the intervention of multiprofessional or multidisciplinary palliative care teams *per se*. Indeed, it is clear from many studies that for most patients, the palliative care team equates to interventions by a doctor and a nurse, often quite separately. Gysel and Higginson perceptively comment that 'more work is needed to test the specific components of palliative care activity and to discover if a different skill mix or interventions performed by the team, are more effective than each other'. For example, there are no studies comparing the efficacy of a well-resourced, well-trained and highly skilled clinical nurse specialist with a back-up team of other professionals for consultation with that of a more traditionally conceived multidisciplinary palliative care team.

It may also be true that multidisciplinary teams have developed in part as a result both of shortcomings in the skill base of individual professionals, and a determination on the part of professionals to hold on to and reinforce the boundaries that determine and create their power. The barriers to good care created by longstanding difficulties in the interface between doctors and nurses are well documented (Finlay 1989). As we move forward, it will be important to assess the impact on practice of recent initiatives such as nurse prescribing, nurse consultants and community matrons. McGrath's careful study (1991) of multiprofessional teamwork amongst community mental handicap teams is clear about the potential problems teamwork brings, as well as its benefits; conflict, time wasting, blurred responsibility, user confusion and increased social control of users. Sadly the NICE report (2004) may inadvertently promote increasing professional stratification and separation through its insistence on distinct, largely professionally dictated competencies for different levels of problem-orientated assessment and referral. Teams can be both fulfilling and frustrating.

For the patient himself, the concept of the multidisciplinary palliative care team may be a very vague one. The team as self-identified may be very different from the team as experienced by the patient. It is the self-identified team that often also identifies and selects the components of the team that it deems necessary for the individual patient. The 'core' multidisciplinary team will also vary in the extent of its inclusion of meeting and communication with more peripheral members of the external team such as the general practitioner (GP), District Nurse, and so on. An element of service rationing has always been implicit in the team allocation and delivery of resources in palliative care. It remains rare that patients are made fully aware of the menu of service and professional offerings available and asked to select their own team package. Patient surveys, such as that undertaken in 1996 by the National Cancer Alliance, do not indicate an overwhelming user demand for multiprofessional teams; they indicate rather that patients want timely care  that is respectful, with coordination and continuity and that provides good physical and medical care in addition to sensitivity and responsiveness to psychological and spiritual issues; which might of course be provided by a well-functioning multidisciplinary team. In reality, patients sometimes complain of the burden of multiple history repetitions to different professionals and of the gaps in communication between such professionals and in the network of care provided. As Monroe (2004a) suggests, what matters is the definition and delivery of the task and not the allocation of a particular role to a particular discipline (see Chapter 2 of this volume). Patients reveal problems to people they trust, and their everyday behaviour reveals their preference for that selected individual to be able to support them in problem management.

One of the most thorough recent studies of multiprofessional team working in health care examined 500 UK general community health care teams and determined four elements vital to successful outcomes: clear objectives, support for innovation, commitment to quality and participation (Borril *et al.* 2001). Borril's work suggested that primary health care teams where professional groups worked together to use their alternative perspectives to generate new knowledge (Opie 2000) delivered higher quality patient care and implemented more innovations. Indeed, Borril concluded that 'the best and most cost effective outcomes for patients and clients are achieved when professionals work together, learn together, engage in clinical audit of outcomes together and generate innovation to ensure progress in practice and service', as evidenced in other chapters of this book. It is theoretically possible to measure whether the necessary conditions for effective teamwork are in place; Borril's study contains many examples of appropriate questionnaires. There has been considerable attention in the literature to the importance of team building;

perhaps the ensuing emphasis on group dynamics (Belbin 1981) has deflected attention from the primary task. However, as we see in Chapter 7 of this volume, a key purpose in focusing on the dynamics within the team is to ensure that the team does not get diverted into 'off task' activity. Katzenbach and Smith's work (1993) suggests that although team building has a positive impact on colleagues' perceptions of one another, it does not increase performance. Guzzo and Shea (1992) assert that teams are energized into effective action by the establishment of significant performance challenges.

In health care inspection and assessment, the emphasis tends to be on process rather than outcomes. Outputs can be measured with relative ease. It is possible, for example, to measure the number of communications with external team members generated by a self-defined team, the number of patients seen, the number of consultations, waiting time from referral to first appointment, rates of emergency hospital admissions, numbers of home deaths, complaints and clinical incidents, the frequency and regularity of team meetings, and whether they are recorded and decisions clearly allocated. The list is endless and is often driven by professional- rather than patient-led agendas. Although some performance management on this kind of basis is undertaken in multiprofessional palliative care teams, the setting and measurement of clear expected outcomes is rarer. There are significant problems in doing so. Outcome measurement has not been a priority in palliative care; existing scales are crude and often focus more on efficacy in pain and symptom control than psychological and social issues. Quality of life scales remain clinically dominated, and more work is needed on measures that allow patients to nominate issues that are important to them rather than simply responding to items chosen by professional teams or researchers (Ahmedzai and Hunt 2004). Another problem is the reliance of many user surveys and regularly administered questionnaires on carer and family member reports, despite evidence that informal and professional carers are poor proxies for individual patient perspectives on need and acceptable outcomes (Heaven and McGuire 1997; Hinton 1994, 1996). Questionnaires about services also often focus on satisfaction with the work of particular professionals rather the efforts of the team. Of course, the decision about outcomes to be measured inevitably varies according to the perspective of the 'owner'. Are the outcomes decided by, or the responses sought from, the team itself, the organization, the purchaser of services, external stakeholders such as GPs, or the service user?

An important component in the efficacy and quality of care and services delivered to patients and families will be the efficacy (skill, knowledge and personal resilience) of the individual delivering the services. As Kahn (2005) reminds us, in caring organizations, technical and emotional work are intertwined and care is delivered partly through the 'technology' of personal relationships. It is important, therefore, that attention is paid to appropriate staff support (Monroe 2004b; see Chapter 7 of this volume). There is some evidence that teams have a buffering effect on the stresses associated with working with death, dying and individual patients through the social support they can provide (Vachon 1995; Rafferty *et al.* 2001). I am unaware of any comparison studies between this effect and the impact of appropriate clinical supervision, which has been slow to take root in medically driven health care environments and which is a well-evaluated vehicle for undertaking the process of active and managed reflection on objectives and tasks (Dunn and Bishop 1998; Gilmore 1999). However, in some of the literature which reviews the experience of nursing staff who have adopted clinical supervision, it is reported that nurses consistently value the provision of 'support' through supervision as a positive and worthwhile experience (see Chapter 7 of this volume; and Butterworth *et al.* 1996; Scanlon and Weir 1997).

Specialist palliative care has traditionally tended to ignore issues of cost effectiveness. These will be significant drivers in the new NHS payment by results contracts. Quality and value for money are now dual goals not alternatives (Bevan 2005). Managing cost effectiveness will inevitably call into question the routine delivery of palliative care by multiprofessional or interdisciplinary teams, and we have to be ready to meet the challenges this will present.

The concept of teamwork in palliative care is deeply entrenched, as are professionally driven agendas, despite the stated emphasis on patient autonomy (Randall and Downie 1999). The dialogue of the hospice movement (characterized by Randall and Downie as 'a cosy shared belief system') has tended to be internal and self-referential, making it difficult to challenge existing practices. In a necessarily resource-strapped future, there will be greater attention paid to creating partnerships with external agencies and an increased focus on cost effectiveness. Demographic and health-related changes mean that most people will die older, suffering multiple chronic illnesses with fewer professional or informal carers to support them. The trend dictated both by individual choice and rational resource allocation is towards support in the community. In this environment, the multiprofessional team may be less appropriate. The inexorable trend will be towards the standard palliative care package being delivered by well-resourced, multi-skilled, individual professionals, most often clinical nurse specialists, who have access to a team of experts for consultation. One of the challenges for the future is how to recruit and train such individuals in addition to focusing attention on the competencies of individual professional members of multi-professional teams. Furthermore, professionals outside the primary base of nursing will need to be trained in the skills of consultancy and in training others in the knowledge and skill base of their own discipline, rather than necessarily as primary interventionists themselves. Looser 'teams' of professionals with different skill and knowledge bases may continue to exist in larger in-patient settings, but cost effectiveness will dictate that their skills in terms of both direct service delivery and consultation will be shared with many institutions rather than just their hub organization. Multiprofessional teams differ in their composition even within a single organization (Payne and Oliviere 2006). In the future, a social worker, art therapist, physiotherapist or chaplain employed by a voluntary hospice may also deliver services to an NHS hospital and to local nursing homes and health centres. Projects along these lines are already taking place. Professional isolation can be avoided and good continuing professional development ensured by a hub and spoke model which allows individuals to train together and to receive clinical supervision and case review in groups based on an appropriate and alternating mixture of uni- and multiprofessional events. Given developing evidence that multi-professional education at all stages of a professional career enhances cooper-ation and coordination in health care delivery as well as encouraging lateral thinking and improved communication, it seems obvious that in the future more attention will be paid to developing such programmes and to developing leaders with appropriate skills to lead (Wee *et al.* 2001; Koffman 2001; Koffman and Higginson 2005).

## What of the future?

If the goal of good end-of-life care for all is to be met, palliative care profes-sionals will need to extend their concept of appropriate team membership to include the wider communities in which patients and those close to them live and work in a more public health approach to palliative care. Given recent societal, demographic and health care changes, it is increasingly clear that formal care services will not be able to meet the needs and demands of all dying and bereaved individuals. Palliative care professionals will need to transfer skills and knowledge to enable both generalist professionals such as teachers and the police, and work colleagues, community groups, friends and neighbours to respond sensitively and appropriately to the needs of the dying and the bereaved. This will be given added impetus as specialist palliative care is encouraged to share and develop its services to non-cancer patients.

A health promotion approach (International Work Group on Death, Dying and Bereavement 2005; Kellehear 2005) can enhance community capacity and resilience. Perhaps we shall then bring into being the until now mostly talked about seamless partnerships between users and professionals. For we are truly one community. We will all die. We will all experience bereavement. The insights of multi- and interdisciplinary teams have helped us to understand the complexity of our differing experiences; the challenge now is to find the most effective way of supporting both those who provide and those who seek palliative care in the future.

# References

Ahmedzai SH and Hunt J (2003). Quality issues in palliative care and supportive care. In: Monroe B and Oliviere D, ed. *Patient Participation in Palliative Care: A Voice for the Voiceless*. Oxford University Press, Oxford. pp. 39–61.

Belbin RM (1981). *Management Teams: Why They Succeed or Fail*. Heinemann, London.

Bevan H (2005). On top-10 lists. *Health Service Journal* 5 May, p. 25.

Borril CS, Carletta J, Carter CS, Dawson JF, Garrod S, Rees A, Richards A, Shapiro D and West MA (2001). *The Effectiveness of HealthCare Teams in the National Health Service*. http://homepages.inf.ed.ac.uk/jeanc/DOH-final-report.pdf

Butterworth T, Bishop V and Carson J (1996). First steps towards evaluating clinical supervision in nursing and health visiting. Part 1: theory, policy and practice development. *Journal of Clinical Nursing* 5, 127–132.

Clark D (2002). *Cicely Saunders. Selected Letters 1959–1999*. Oxford University Press, Oxford.

Department of Health (1998). *A First Class Service. Quality in the New NHS*. Stationery Office, London.

Dunn C and Bishop V (1998). Clinical supervision: its implementation in one acute sector trust. In: Bishop V, ed. *Clinical Supervision in Practice*. Macmillan, London, pp. 85–107.

Ellershaw JE, Peat SJ and Boys LC (1995). Assessing the effectiveness of a hospital palliative care team. *Palliative Medicine* 9, 145–152.

Finlay I (1989). Sources of stress in hospice medical directors and matrons. *Palliative Medicine* 4, 5–9.

Gilmore A (1999). *Review of U.K. Evaluative Literature on Clinical Supervision in Nursing and Health Visiting*. UKCC, London.

Guzzo RA, Shea GP, Dunnette MD, Hough LM, eds (1992). *Handbook of Industrial and Organisational Psychology*. Consulting Psychologists Press, Palo Alto, CA. p. 269.

Gysels M and Higginson IJ (2004). *Improving Supportive and Palliative Care for Adults With Cancer: Research Evidence Manual*. National Institute for Clinical Excellence, London.

Hearn JH and Higginson IJ (1998). Do specialist palliative care teams improve outcomes for cancer patients? A systematic review. *Palliative Medicine* 12, 317–332.

Heaven CM and Maguire P (1997). Disclosure of concerns by hospice patients and their identification by nurses. *Palliative Medicine* 11, 283–290.

Hinton J (1994). Can home care maintain an acceptable quality of life for patients with terminal cancer and their relatives? *Palliative Medicine,* 8, 183–196.

Hinton J (1996). Services given and help perceived during home care for terminal cancer. *Palliative Medicine* 10, 125–135.

International Work Group on Death, Dying and Bereavement (2005). Charter for the Normalisation of Dying, Death and Loss. Draft statement. *Mortality,* 10, 157–161.

Kahn WA (2005). *Holding Fast—The Struggle to Create Resilient Organisations*. Brunner Routledge, Hove, UK.

Katzenbach JR and Smith KS (1993). The wisdom of teams. In: *Why Teams?* Harvard Business School, Boston, MA, pp. 11–14.

Kellehear A (2005). *Compassionate Cities. Public Health and End of Life Care*. Routledge, London.

Koffman J (2001). Multiprofessional palliative care education: past challenges, future issues. *Journal of Palliative Care* 17, 86–92.

Koffman J and Higginson IJ (2005). Assessing the effectiveness and acceptability of interprofessional palliative care education. *Journal of Palliative Care* 21, 262–269.

McGrath M (1991). *Multi-disciplinary Teams*. Gower, Aldershot, UK.

Monroe, B (2004a). Social work in palliative care. In: Doyle D, Hanks G and Cherny NI, ed. *Oxford Textbook of Palliative Medicine*, 3rd edn. Oxford University Press, Oxford, pp. 1005–1018.

Monroe B. (2004b). Emotional impact of palliative care on staff. In: Sykes N, Edmonds P and Wiles J, ed. *Management of Advanced Disease*, 4th edn. Edward Arnold, London, pp. 450–460.

National Cancer Alliance. (1996). *Patient-centred Cancer Services? What Patients Say*. National Cancer Alliance, Oxford.

NICE (2004). *Guidance on Cancer Services: Improving Supportive and Palliative Care for Adults with Cancer*. National Institute for Clinical Excellence, London.

Opie A (2000). *Thinking Teams/Thinking Clients: Knowledge-based Teamwork*. Columbia University Press, New York.

Payne M and Oliviere D (2006). The interdisciplinary team. In: Walsh D, ed. *Palliative Medicine*. Elsevier, New York (in press).

Rafferty AM, Ball J and Aiken LH (2001). Are teamwork and professional autonomy compatible, and do they result in improved hospital care? *Quality in Health Care* 10 (Suppl II), 32–37.

Randall F and Downie RS (1999). *Palliative Care Ethics. A Companion for all Specialities*, 2nd edn. Oxford University Press, Oxford.

Scanlon C and Weir WS (1997). Learning from practice? Mental health nurses perceptions and experiences of clinical supervision. *Journal of Advanced Nursing* 26, 295–303.

Vachon M (1995). Staff stress in hospice/palliative care: a review. *Palliative Medicine* 9, 91–122.

Wee B, Hillier R, Coles C, Mountford B, Sheldon F and Turner P. (2001). Palliative care: a suitable setting for undergraduate interprofessional education. *Palliative Medicine* 15, 487–492.

Zwarenstein M and Bryant W (2000). Interventions to improve collaboration between nurses and doctors. In: Bero L, Grilli R, Grimshaw J, Oxman A and Zwarenstein M, ed. Cochrane Collaboration on effective professional practice module of the Cochrane database of systematic reviews. *Cochrane Library*. Issue 2. Oxford (update software 2000).

Zwarenstein M and Reeves S (2000). What's so great about collaboration? Editorial. *British Medical Journal* 320, 1022–1023.

# 14

# Conclusion

*Peter Speck*

This book has focused on a variety of aspects of teamwork within the field of palliative care. The development of most teams has been an evolutionary process. This has been dictated by the availability of people with vision and commitment to palliative care, the availability of finance, a variety of settings in which to be located, and a willingness of professionals and users to explore together creative ways of working and offering a service—all of which have contributed to the shaping of teams.

In exploring the differences between a group and a team within this book, it is clear that focusing on, and owning, a shared common task is fundamental to team development. The membership of teams in palliative care varies in size and composition, and the multidisciplinary nature of most teams has been examined, together with the need to ensure that the user voice is adequately represented and heard. There has deliberately been no analysis of the role undertaken by each discipline represented within the team. This is because each person will take up their role in a variety of ways, as they think best enables the team as a whole to fulfil the primary task of the unit or team. Within any profession, individuals will adopt a variety of styles of working and, if they feel secure within their professional identity, will be able to incorporate a degree of flexibility in the way in which they fulfil their role within the team. What is important in respect of the different roles occupied by people is that the leadership ensures there is discussion and clarification about expectations of the different team members. If the expectations of people (in terms of duties and obligations) are not clear, then ambiguity will develop and eventually lead to role conflict. Unclear expectations are a great source of conflict and stress within a team and often lead to people taking on inappropriate tasks and becoming overloaded, or losing sight of their primary task. As the team moves to a more interdisciplinary way of working, these issues become more important in order to enable each member to contribute effectively. For example, a chaplain or spiritual care provider may adopt a wider role than solely the provision of religious ritual because of the skills she/ he possesses, the needs of the team, and a view of spirituality that is wider than religious expression. If the chaplain is labelled as the religious provider and stereotyping occurs, it might become difficult for the chaplain to make a wider contribution to the team by drawing on other insights into the needs and responses of the patient, family and staff. The ability to manage 'difference' is a core skill for interdisciplinary working as it allows members to avoid stereo-typical behaviour and acting on assumptions. Instead they can explore together their different understanding of roles held within the team and the opportunities these present for creative working.

The ways in which the users, and the stakeholders' voices are listened to will also reflect the degree of security members feel in both their professional identity and their role. A great deal hinges on the ability of the leader to lead and the individual's style of leadership. Power and powerlessness feature strongly in health care settings and lead to a variety of tensions within a team, and between teams, or the organization in which they are located. At one end of the spectrum, the individual members of a team can feel empowered to do the work they are there to do and to cooperate with col-leagues and users within and outside of the team. At the other end, they can experience the effects of people who misuse their power and seek to control or bully those who are 'different' from themselves, or of a different professional group. Once again the leader of the palliative care team needs to be aware of the issues being faced by team members as they go around the hospice or hospital, or into the community. Good communication and negotiating skills can enable effective team working as well as collaboration between teams, to say nothing of the therapeutic relationship with patients and carers.

We have acknowledged that teams do not just happen, neither do they continue to thrive, and remain fulfilling, unless there is appropriate attention paid to 'process' and the team dynamic. This can occur as part of training in that, if training is undertaken in a multidisciplinary way, it can help to foster good relationships and challenge some of the stereotypes and assumptions we may have about professions other than our own. It can also help us to develop a better understanding of the language or jargon used within different discip-lines which can become very confusing, if not irritating, in team meetings. Team building is another focus for looking at how a team develops and how change might be addressed. The point is made earlier (Chapter 8) that while a specific activity such as an 'away day' may be useful, team building activities should be a regular part of the ongoing life of the team. Much of this should happen informally and not just as a result of some specific event or structured activity.

A similar point is made in respect of addressing team dynamics and ensuring appropriate support for those engaged in palliative care. The observational study of life in a palliative care unit indicated clearly how people can be affected by the nature of what they are engaged in. To maintain a healthy team involves ensuring that 'process', and unconscious processes in particular, are not ignored. Whether the team is located in one place (such as an in-patient unit) or scattered over a wide geographical area, it is important that some time is given to asking questions such as 'How do you feel the team is functioning at present?' or 'How are people feeling. Are there any issues relating to us here, or other teams, that we need to discuss?' 'Are there any particular patients or families that are affecting us and proving stressful?' One aspect of a healthy team is its ability to ask the 'unaskable' questions, to speak the 'unspeakable' and work with any discomfort this creates. Often dynamic issues can be explored together by the team members if there is a sufficient degree of trust and respect for each other, and confidentiality is assured. Sometimes it may be beneficial to invite an outside facilitator to meet with the team to enable these issues to be looked at and free the leader to participate as a member. Where the team is working on different sites, or not able to meet together very often, it may be that part of a meeting for another purpose (e.g. clinical supervision, case review or update) may need to be set aside for such a focus. This is not wasteful 'navel-gazing' but an essential ingredient for team well-being, though it should not dominate the life of the team and become an 'off task' activity.

Palliative care teams do not exist in isolation and, in addition to their relationship with the NHS and/or charitable body, they also are located within a society in which they live as well as work. This means that advances in what medical science can achieve can lead to an expansion in the ethical dimension of the work. The specialist palliative care team will be expected to have, or have access to, specialist knowledge of the ethical dilemmas associated with end-of-life care and be able to contribute to patient, family and clinical colleague enquiries for advice. Whether working in isolation or as part of a cohesive team, those working in palliative care will continue to wrestle with the tension arising from the interplay between personal values and the espoused values of palliative care as well as the values of the team. Linked to this is the legal framework in which we work. The closer we move towards a more interdisciplinary style of working, the more important it is to be aware of this legal dimension. Issues such as accountability, liability, confidentiality and the principles of malpractice all have a legal as well as an ethical and managerial aspect to them, and need to receive due attention in any health care team comprising different professional and non-professional people. It is interesting to note Montgomery's comment that 'by fixing the standard of care according to the post that people take within the team, the law reinforces the mutual interdependence that characterizes good teamwork' (Chapter 12).

In the current climate of further change within the UK NHS, it is clear that we need to recognize that more teams will operate away from in-patient units as there develops a greater emphasis on care in the community. This is something very familiar in many other parts of the world where, financially, it is often not possible to build a UK-style in-patient hospice. As the provision of care develops a greater emphasis on community care, it is likely that membership of teams in the future may include a variety of non-health care providers. This carries with it the danger that the team could fragment into a group, with implications for leadership and the task being addressed. If the patient and family are to experience continuity of care from diagnosis to death, there will need to be good collaborative working and coordination of the different inputs, or the care provision may begin to unravel. There have been several examples in the UK press of multiagency family involvement where the care offered to client or patient has failed because of poor communication or lack of effective liaison between service providers. While a clearly defined interdisciplinary team approach may be more difficult to achieve and maintain, I believe that the principles of such an approach will still need to be applied.

Thus, the group of caregivers concerned must have an agreed common task or aim and have a shared ownership in trying to achieve that aim. They also need to acknowledge their interdependence if quality care is to be delivered. The prime importance of clear communication between all of those involved cannot be overemphasized, and the patient and family as well as other community workers need to be included. Whatever the future structures for delivering palliative care may be like, there will still need to be effective leadership, both to build and support the team and to ensure continuity of care for the users. Expectations and accountability must be clear to all concerned, with appropriate attention to process and outcomes. Once you begin to talk in these terms, you are once again describing teamwork.

Competitiveness between agencies and service providers can erode the necessary trust, respect and collaboration required, and before effective teamwork can evolve some unlearning of old ways of relating and working together in the light of new circumstances may need to happen. Wilson sums this up well:

The principles of teamworking may be easily understood, but the task of installing it can be quite daunting. Introducing teamworking is not a straightforward grafting job, the simple matter of adding a new idea to those already in place. It is about making a fundamental change in the way people work. Every teamworking application is different. Each organisation, department and individual group is faced with unique problems and in some situations it is more about getting rid of old ways of doing things than injecting new ones (Wilson 1998).

The future may hold a great deal of uncertainty about how palliative care will best be provided and resourced in both the UK and elsewhere. Patients with non-malignant disease as well as those with malignancies will look to palliative care for alleviation of physical, psycho-social and spiritual needs, and distress. If greater patient choice in the place of care can be achieved, more may chose a hospice rather than hospital with possible increased demand for in-patient and community care. The scope is enormous. One of the main challenges will be to adapt the tenets of good team working to changing patterns of health care provision, in collaboration with the users of services, and to resource and enable other care teams to enhance their own palliative and end-of-life care.

It has been important to reflect on the effectiveness of teamwork because we should be able to articulate and demonstrate why we believe that Team 'X' is a well-functioning, effective and healthy team. It remains surprising that there is so little empirical evidence to show that satisfactory outcomes are (or are not) related to team-as-a-whole interventions, rather than by a well-resourced individual with a good back-up team. Quantitative approaches to efficacy need to be supplemented with newly developed qualitative methods. We may be able to describe the number of visits made, the number of days spent in in-patient care and the cost of interventions, but what of the quality of the care given, the satisfaction felt. If the patient or family express good satisfaction with the care they have received, is that related to a resourceful individual, or to an individual representative of a well-functioning resourceful team? Teams should not be created simply because they are considered to be a good idea. To echo Farsides in re-phrasing Kant (Chapter 11) 'A team is a means to an end, as opposed to being an end in itself'. There is, I believe, a research need for studies to investigate the benefits of interdisciplinary team input versus that of a well-resourced individual. We also need to investigate what users would choose as their 'team of choice', given a clear idea of the various resources that could be made available to them, at various points of the patient journey.

After working for >30 years in a variety of teams, in a variety of roles, I believe teams do enable us to provide the opportunity to develop the integrated, seamless, service many espouse to. Their effectiveness in caring for patients and carers, and providing a healthy balance between frustration and fulfilment for members, will depend largely on clear leadership, commitment to each other and to the task. That task is not some organizational/managerial statement but person-centred care. Above all, team working should enable us to maintain our focus on the person cared for, as well as affirming our own humanity.

The song writer and singer Paul McCartney said:

I love to hear a choir. I love the humanity... to see the faces of real people devoting themselves to a piece of music. I like the teamwork. It makes me feel optimistic about the human race when I see them cooperating like that.

## References

McCartney P. http://en.thinkexist.com/services/bookmark.asp?id=256545&quote=i_love_to_hear_a...

Wilson J (1998). Building teams—with attitude. *Professional Manager* September, p. 13.

# Index

Note to index: page numbers in bold indicate tables